Pathologies of Patriarchy

Pathologies of Patriarchy

Death, Suffering, Care, and Coping in the Gendered Gaps of HIV/AIDS Interventions in Nigeria

Eloho Ese Basikoro

ROWMAN &
LITTLEFIELD
INTERNATIONAL
London • New York

Published by Rowman & Littlefield International Ltd
6 Tinworth Street, London, SE11 5AL, UK
www.rowmaninternational.com

Rowman & Littlefield International Ltd. is an affiliate of Rowman & Littlefield

4501 Forbes Boulevard, Suite 200, Lanham, Maryland 20706, USA
With additional offices in Boulder, New York, Toronto (Canada), and Plymouth (UK)
www.rowman.com

British Library Cataloguing in Publication Data
A catalogue record for this book is available from the British Library

ISBN: HB 978-1-78660-770-6

Library of Congress Cataloging-in-Publication Data Is Available

ISBN 978-1-78660-770-6 (cloth: alk. paper)
ISBN 978-1-78660-771-3 (electronic)

Contents

Acknowledgments

I give thanks to God Almighty whom I serve because I could never have written this book or conducted the research that informed this book without His extraordinary grace, and for the many times I thought I would give up and could no longer push beyond what I thought was the end of myself, I found amazing inner strength through Him.

I also owe gratitude to a community of individuals, who have provided me intellectual, moral, and spiritual support in the course of this book and its research. This book is a product of my dissertation research, conducted with the support of a great committee of professors at the Geography Department, University of Washington, Seattle. I am indeed very fortunate to have had Professors Matthew Sparke, Lucy Jarosz, and Jonathan Mayer as my advisory committee and for their moral and intellectual support in the initial research and writing process that culminated in this book. At the University of Washington, my sincere thanks also go to the Geography Department, and the African Studies Program at the Henry M. Jackson School of International Studies, for the funds awarded to me to support the conduct of this research, through the Howard Martins and Ottenberg-Winans African Studies fellowships respectively.

In 2016, I met Holly Tyler through the American Association of Geographers' conference, the commissioning editor at Rowman and Littlefield International Press at the time, who believed in the timeliness and significance of this research, and offered me the opportunity to publish this work as a book. I think my meeting with Holly was timely because I was at the crossroads of making a career-changing decision, whether to continue in academia or to transition into the nonacademic sector. Holly's proposal sealed the deal for me as I accepted the opportunity to publish my dissertation research as a book but which also meant that this research may not be making it into published journal articles in line with pursuing a career in academia. I am also grateful to her for the support she rendered me at the proposal stage of this book project.

I also want to acknowledge and thank Archbishop Goddowell Awomakpa for his care and support, and who also provided great accommodation and transportation for my husband and me during our four months stay in Nigeria for the research work. Great gratitude also goes to Mrs. Otebele, the hospital administrator at the HIV treatment facility in Erhoike, who gave me the opportunity to talk with the healthcare workers and other research participants, in particular, the women living with HIV who were so kind and gracious to have given me their time and stories. It is to them that I dedicate this book. Their strength, resilience, and hope amid their ongoing struggle—confronting the everyday challenges of living with HIV as women in a deeply patriarchal society—have truly inspired me with the grace to write this book so that their voices too can be heard. I also owe many thanks to all the health workers at the treatment facility whom I interviewed, for their time and warm reception to me all the times I visited the facility.

Thanks to Uche and Aghogho Onyebuchi, who provided me access to some policy stakeholders at the national public health sector, whom I may not have otherwise had access to. In the same manner, I give my thanks to all the policy stakeholders whom I interviewed at the National Agency for the Control of AIDS and Federal Ministry of Health, Abuja, as well as stakeholders in the nongovernmental organizations, in Benin and Abuja, whose names I cannot mention here because of researcher-participant confidentiality.

To Adaeze Agbaje and her family, many thanks to them for opening their home to me for the period I was in Abuja, conducting the policy stakeholders' interviews. Very special thanks to my professors, friends, and colleagues, Lucy Jarosz, Michael Olu Adediran, Todd Faubion, Mónica Farías, Donald Edokpa, Glory Enarubve, Ronnie Thibault, Ese Akpede, and Rev. Fr. Felix Odobi, who provided great feedback on each chapter of this book, believed in its significance and timeliness, and told me so in not very few words. Thanks also to my spiritual directors, Pastor Tiveh Elijah Odjuvwuederie and Rev. Fr. Daniel Oghenerukevwe, for their spiritual and moral support.

My thanks and appreciation also go to my parents, Michael and Magdalene Tobrise, for their love, consistent prayers, moral support, and encouragement. I am so proud to have you both as my parents and will always remain grateful for the foundation you laid for me, without which I will not be the person I am today. I acknowledge all of my siblings, especially Efetobore Anita Tobrise, for constantly checking in with me about my writing progress. Last but certainly not least, I acknowledge my spouse, Anthony Basikoro. You have always believed in me and affirmed my abilities even in moments of self-doubt. My frequent intellectual debates with you helped immensely to shape this work especially at the dissertation level. You have stayed by me through the highs and lows of this journey from the beginning to the end, and your faith in me kept me strong because I wanted to do you proud. I owe you many thanks!

Part 1

HISTORY, POLITICS, AND HIV/AIDS GOVERNANCE

Chapter 1

Gender, HIV/AIDS, and Treatment Sustainability

In many sub-Saharan African countries, HIV-seropositive women intentionally shun life-saving medical technologies like antiretroviral (ARV) drugs or only engage inconsistently with treatment regimens.[1] An obvious contradiction in these spaces has been the limited, uneven, and inconsistent access to treatment by HIV-seropositive women, with direct implications for adherence and retention in care. Poor patterns of ARV access and self-destructive behaviors of nonadherence continue in this spatial context despite the free provision of drugs in some geographies and institutional policies that claim to be inclusive of the needs of HIV-seropositive patients.[2] Such paradoxical patterns demand urgent attention and this book's main aim is to provide context on how and why these patterns persist. It does so based on close ethnographic investigation of the social contexts, and associated constraints and inequalities delimiting the ways women living with HIV (WLWH)[3] access and experience biomedical treatment regimens. As such, a fundamental proposition that underpins the arguments that this book makes is that orthodox biomedical analyses of interventions fall short insofar as they elide the social realities of vulnerable women, with methods that assume too much about these women's experiences of treatment. While a purely biomedical model may be vital for deploying effective health solutions, it becomes inadequate in realms where social forces and structural violence strongly mediate individual and group experiences of health like much of the spaces in sub-Saharan Africa. In the words of renowned medical anthropologist, Paul Farmer:

> Structural violence is one way of describing social arrangements that put individuals and populations in harm's way. The arrangements are structural because they are embedded in the political and economic organization of our social

> world; they are violent because they cause injury to people . . . neither culture nor pure individual will is at fault; rather, historically given (and often economically driven) processes and forces conspire to constrain individual agency. Structural violence is visited upon all those whose social status denies them access to the fruits of scientific and social progress.[4]

Such violence, in turn, structures and strictures individual agency, thus, radically limiting the options of vulnerable populations such as women.[5] In these structured and strictured spaces, health outcomes are rarely singular products of biological causation. Rather, they are an interaction of a multiplicity of macro- and micro-factors that are also socioeconomic, political, and cultural but intricately interwoven and transcending epidemiological understandings.[6] This is the overall premise of this book and further claims build logically from this key proposition.

In challenging orthodox biomedical interventions that elide the social realities of vulnerable populations and reductionist methods that oversimplify women's experiences of treatment, I situate this HIV treatment discourse within a health and development framework. This is in conjunction with a broad focus on the political economy to foreground the intricate ways that issues around gender at the level of the body are constituted and enacted under the influence of global-local structural ties and tensions. In this regard, this book's authority and value are also premised on its foundations in embodied gender research into the socio-geographical complexities of HIV treatment access and adherence. Consequently, a core theme that I recurrently engage in this book is the *relationality of scale*—a term deployed by feminist political geographer, Caroline Faria, to describe how the female body is positioned and bound in an intricate web of social, economic, and political relations in different spaces and across multiples scales.[7] And I deploy the concept of gender in this book using Michael Kevane's definition, which is gender as "the constellation of rules and identities that prescribe and proscribe behavior for persons, in their social roles as men and women. These rules and identities may be deliberate or unintended, explicit or implicit, conscious or unconscious."[8] Although I frame gender broadly as constitutive of women and men as they are in relation with each other, throughout this book, the analytical focus will be on women (in particular, HIV-seropositive women) because of the ways that patriarchal power has acted to feminize the HIV/AIDS epidemic and continues to reproduce the inequalities that disempower women in their access to HIV/AIDS biomedical interventions.[9]

A key situation at stake is also that of the household, a space that is especially an important site of struggle in gendered power relations. One of the claims that I make in this book is that unsustained HIV treatment access among WLWH occurs at the intersection of two seemingly contradictory scales—the personal and the structural—yet these are mutually connected and reinforcing. The fundamental argument that the intimate is always global has never been truer in the individual experiences of HIV/AIDS, which though ostensibly border on individual behavior and underpinned by the relations of power at the level of the household, are primarily mediated by broader forces operating at various scales of influence which determine the power of individual choice.[10] In many contexts, legal and formal unions like marriage form the basis of a household. However, in representing a variety of social, cultural, legal, and political systems, less formal unions like cohabitation also form the basis of family life and the household. Based on the sociocultural context of the geography in reference, this book's definition of the household entails formal unions like marriage, and informal consensual unions based on cohabitation as well as polygyny, for example, where a man takes more than one wife.[11]

Like the diverse connections that Mark Hunter's *Love in the Time of AIDS* makes between the political economy and the gendered intimate experiences of everyday life of people in the South African HIV/AIDS epidemic using a historical and socio-geographical perspective, this book also adopts this approach to situate the pathologies of HIV/AIDS and the response of development agencies but within the broad interactions of patriarchy, environmental change, and the global political economy of aid.[12] In this sense, my models of analysis also come from other geographers as well as anthropologists.[13] The analysis also illuminates the intricate ways that these myriad forces have shaped the local landscape of HIV treatment interventions in Nigeria.

This book also makes an important distinction because it moves away from the recurrent emphasis on the political, social, and cultural causes of the sub-Saharan African HIV/AIDS epidemic. While the analysis touches on these foundations to provide the needed background to contextualize the pathology and experience of the disease, at its core, this book brings an explicit treatment perspective especially to those who are interested in how the material, sociocultural, and political dynamics of causation around the disease are reproduced in intervention efforts, particularly in HIV therapeutic regimens, and in the current disposition where treatment is valued as the new preventative mechanism.

The geography of HIV/AIDS in sub-Saharan Africa mirrors spaces of individual and group vulnerabilities to risk whether this is referenced within a causal, preventative, or treatment framework. To illuminate the intricate details of the HIV/AIDS experience in particular places is to adopt an epistemology that gives recognition to the nuances of place as determinants of health behavior and outcomes. Hence, health geography forms the dominant epistemology for this research because it stresses the study of health and health care within broader biosocial models using more interpretive methods, with an awareness of the active role of place in shaping health.[14] Health geographers construct health and health outcomes as transcending an essentialized disease and biomedical paradigm, to including social forces, and also as products of the complex interactions of place processes and relations.[15]

Situated in Erhoike, an oil-producing community in the oil-rich Niger Delta region of Nigeria, the analysis presented in this book constructs the personal treatment experiences of HIV-seropositive women within a wider matrix of the oil economy and its associated complexities, including violence, conflicts, resource control, distribution, and access, and the ways these constrain available opportunities for women, and by implication, health decision-making.[16] Of particular importance is that this discursive analysis of environmental change processes elucidates the role of global capitalist configurations by transnational oil policies and their investments on local environments and social systems in third world geographies, acting through the apparatuses of national and domestic policies to impact locally on vulnerable bodies.[17] Using an intersectional lens, this book uncovers this convoluted web of social, cultural, political, geographical, and institutional arrangements as they are deeply entangled in the gendering of treatment access and adherence among twenty-two HIV-seropositive women living in the Niger Delta region—faced with intense suffering from stigma, rejection, abandonment, and poverty—and in turn, the ways that treatment becomes embodied at these intersections.

Amid all these intersections, gender is crucial in coming to terms with HIV treatment inequalities. The testimonials of HIV-seropositive women that are narrated in this book are intended to give agency to the voice of a group of women who are central in development, yet mostly silent in its theory and practice, and to produce what Donna Haraway has famously described as location-specific or *situated knowledges*.[18] The rationale underpinning the production of location-specific knowledge is to represent with more exactness the ways that the local, state, and global economies of power become causal mechanisms that position women's bodies as spaces of risk and vulnerability.[19] This argument connects the intimate to multiple contexts and scales.[20] For example, it links the social, national, and global by explicating how the uneven practices of interventions in the global-local HIV/AIDS landscape and structural processes at a national scale materialize into the local and embodied experiences of women at the personal and household levels. This is not to argue that there are not existing studies that have attempted to link the experience of HIV/AIDS to gender and the political economy. Rather, there have been too many broad generalizations, especially in the sub-Saharan African HIV/AIDS context, with the specific intricacies of everyday life that result from these macro-level interactions in particular geographies less underscored. Such decontextualized connections produce ineffective

HIV/AIDS policies and programs which undermine HIV-seropositive women's access and adherence to treatment and care.

The alternative analyses offered in this book locate HIV-seropositive women's access and adherence to treatment, and their retention in care, across these multiple contextual scales. Across these scales, the persistence of patriarchal social relations is shown to be a dominant influence on health outcomes and a primary cause of pathology, suffering, and premature death. This book offers insights into one of the many paradoxes in HIV/AIDS interventions whereby the very process of treatment that is designed to be life-saving is intentionally shunned by those facing the risk of death.[21]

KEY THEORIES AND CONCEPTS

The idea of the research that underpins this book was influenced by my various identities and interests. As a health geographer and a woman from a minority ethnic group in the Niger Delta region of Nigeria, my own gendered experiences of place shaped by the relations of patriarchy have provided me important perspectives to focus this study. Above my own interest, this book's intention also aims to amplify the outcry and voices of women infected with HIV or suffering from AIDS, in order to foreground their needs and the gender-blind nature of interventions. Needs that are unmet either because of the exclusion of gender as a category of concern in interventions, or because of how, even when included, health services fail to adequately address women's needs.[22]

Like most sub-Saharan African countries, gender inequalities, differential access to health services, and many forms of structural and gender-based violence predispose women to the risks of HIV/AIDS.[23] Yet interventions have remained gender blind as gender considerations are invoked in policy discourses but elided in practice; thus, women continue to be constrained in their uptake of treatment.[24] In Nigeria, the HIV treatment terrain remains an uneven landscape with huge gaps that gender access, adherence, and retention in care.[25] The National Agency for the Control of AIDS (NACA), the main body responsible for coordinating HIV/AIDS interventions in the country, reported an estimated less than 50 percent antiretroviral therapy (ART) coverage among eligible antiretroviral patients—adults and children—as of 2014.[26] Although this report provides no data insight into gender disparities, country assessment reports in Nigeria suggest that women are disproportionately affected in the area of treatment access and care.[27] Despite the less than optimal levels of treatment coverage and access, a recent report by the Joint United Nations Program on HIV/AIDS (UNAIDS) shows a general increase in ART coverage with about 53 percent of adults (15 years and over) living with HIV on treatment as of 2018.[28] Nevertheless, these progressive reports do not always reflect the specific ways that people experience treatment. Rather, they belie the day-to-day experiences of the social and economic inequalities confronted by people living with HIV, and how these affect treatment access and adherence amid universal accessibility to treatment.[29]

But beyond the numbers or rates of those accessing treatment, key questions emerge about the pattern and distribution of treatment, namely, who does treatment include or exclude, who benefits or who is marginalized? These questions remain crucial even in countries like Brazil, Thailand, and Mozambique that have actively pursued universal access to treatment.[30] In turn, these questions underline the vital need to assess discrepancies between universalizing policy ambitions around treatment coverage and exposing ground realities of huge inequalities in access and distribution. This reality necessitates urgent attention to address service gaps that prevent HIV/AIDS communities and individuals from achieving the full health benefits of ARTs. The dearth of information on this topic is one of the many reasons that makes this book imperative and opportune, especially in the light of current global debates on closing the gaps in treatment. Not in the least, is also the need to provide practical perspectives from the field through the lens of HIV subjects and development actors who are key stakeholders in this discourse, and in ways that aim to bridge the gap between theory and practice.

Access and Adherence

Evidently, access and adherence are two recurring terms that I deploy to contextualize HIV-seropositive women's experiences of treatment. It is pertinent, therefore, to clarify how these terms are deployed in this book. Important too is the need to mention that while I engage these constructs as a binary, I observed that the term, access relative to adherence, is less used in the social medical literature on HIV/AIDS. It stands to reason that with improved access to ARTs, there may be a shifting focus from access to an increasing attention on adherence and retention in care. Yet, in practice, these two terms remain mutually constitutive as adherence is contingent on access.

Universal definitions of access are, therefore, not commonplace. For example, a vast body of geographical work largely problematizes and frames access to health services in terms of spatial accessibility; that is, as a function of time, distance, and physical proximity to service locations, with access sometimes abstracted and reduced to the notion of availability which stipulates a very narrow medical focus.[31] But empirical results from this study challenge this conceptualization of access, adding a social and feminist geographical perspective to the ways in which space, and thus access, are simultaneously produced and mediated by gendered inequalities and structural constraints. Access is thus reconceptualized here in terms of systems and practices that either enable or disenable the physical, social, and material agency of health subjects to obtain and effectively utilize health services at will, and in this context, ARV treatment. This definition is constructed from the general framings of ARV access in the geographies of health care and HIV/AIDS literature as well as the direct experiences of women referenced in this book.[32]

A 2013 World Health Organization (WHO) report defines adherence in the context of HIV treatment as "the extent to which a person's behavior—taking medications, following a diet and/or executing lifestyle changes—corresponds with agreed recommendations from a health care provider."[33] By extension, nonadherence is the reverse. In this definition, a provider-patient relationship is emphasized with the onus of responsibility and compliance to treatment tasked on both the provider and the patient respectively. In practice, consultations take place between the provider and the patient, and treatment is commenced contingent on a mutually agreed regimen.[34] In this arrangement, patients are considered active subjects and decision-makers in the treatment process, rather than as passive recipients of medical instructions from a health provider, in order to ensure patient compliance. Although the role of healthcare professionals is emphasized, adherence is very much patient-centric because patients are expected to behave in ways that ensure that treatment outcomes are achieved.[35] While noncompliance can be influenced by a range of clinical factors including drug toxicity and other side effects,[36] biomedical perspectives of nonadherence are overly emphasized with social and material dimensions often neglected or less underscored.

Closely related to adherence is the term retention, which is the "continuous engagement with appropriate medical care."[37] Conversely, lack of retention is the complete disengagement from HIV treatment and care. It is also important to mention that clinical non-retention does not mean a lack of retention in care as patients may discontinue access to ARV treatment in a particular facility but continue to remain in the larger continuum of care, for example, seeking treatment from other health facilities.[38] Although the terms adherence and retention appear synonymous, I draw attention to an important distinction between them. Whereas adherence puts the onus largely on patients to take personal responsibility for their treatment in terms of daily uptake of medication, appropriate dosage, and general medication guidelines, retention shifts most of the responsibility to caregivers and treatment programs through an established monitoring system that ensures that patients remain in care. This appears to be an obvious contradiction because the practice of adherence as mostly a patient-regulated exercise seems to ignore the same situational contexts that may compel infected individuals to drop out of care. This distinction becomes significant in health contexts where ARV noncompliant patients are labeled as defaulters, which feeds into a long-standing cultural politics and HIV/AIDS paradigm—the *blame-the-victim* culture.[39] The distinction between adherence and retention in care is also important in this current era of HIV/AIDS interventions where emphases on self-responsibility through strict adherence messages fail to address the many systemic barriers that HIV-seropositive women have to overcome to maintain their treatment regimen and remain in care.

In this book, I demonstrate what is problematic or at least limited with the language and practice of adherence as mostly an issue of individual responsibility. I make a conscious effort to shift from popular notions that conceptualize treatment access and adherence in over-simplistic and individualistic terms, and that also fail to factor in the external constraints that complicate treatment experiences at the personal level. This argument foregrounds the tension between individual and institutional responsibilities in HIV treatment therapies. It also connects to the overall premise of this book which challenges the erroneous signification of access and adherence to treatment, as well as retention in care through individualized discourses and practices that ignore the broader structures that undermine the personal agency to materialize such responsibilities.

Gender Frames and Positionality

As I mentioned hitherto, my personal gender concerns formed a major premise of this book's underlying research. It also informed the ways that I operationalized the research process—design and methods, the personal decisions I made during the fieldwork, and the ways I negotiated relations with research participants. As I reflect on the fieldwork process, my own gendered experiences in the research sites are a testament to the timeliness and significance of this book and the dire need to reinforce the push for gender equality in Nigeria. Throughout the research process, I was personally aware of my positionality as a woman and also the implication of researching gender issues in a male-dominated society. Such realizations guided the design of the research instruments. For example, in the framing of the interviews and focus group discussion guides, I made an effort to distance myself from the use of words or language that were explicitly associated with the concept of feminism, even though feminist theories form key intellectual perspectives that frame this research. In lieu of this, I deployed the concept of gender equality as this has become a more acceptable phrase, given its wider human rights appeal especially in policy circles. Yet there were times this work was met with resistance by policy stakeholders, mostly men, which calls attention to the fact that the struggle for gender equality in Nigeria is still at its inception.

To illustrate, I attended a policy dissemination conference on gender equality and gender-based violence in Abuja, Nigeria's federal capital territory. At the meeting, a male policy stakeholder who sat beside me remarked about what he described as an excessive focus on gender issues, and the problem of conflating gender with women. He further opined that the issue of gender inequality as it concerns women was overrated and men were beginning to feel marginalized especially in areas they feel a need for empowerment. In another instance, a male policy stakeholder whom I had approached for permission to conduct interviews vehemently questioned my authority to conduct research on gender inequality. He referenced multiple aspects of my identities as antithetical to my authority. He asserted that a researcher from an institution in a Western country should not conduct research on local women in Nigeria, completely eliding the fact that I am not only Nigerian but an indigene of the Niger Delta region which appropriately positioned me for this knowledge process. He also challenged my ethnicity and claimed that as a female researcher from a minority ethnic group, I was weakly positioned to challenge the injustices of gender inequality that my research sought to address. On the contrary, these particular contested identities bring a rich and grounded local perspective to the issues at stake because of my situatedness—as a researcher and woman—in the historically exploited and marginalized Niger Delta region.

Although the claims by this policy maker can be argued as subjective and even biased, they are not in entirety, diametrically opposed to the moral and ethical dilemmas in feminist geographical research which seek to redress colonizing academic praxes that simultaneously legitimize the voices of Western academic scholars and episteme but silence or remarginalize indigenous knowledge and voices in developing world spaces. Also less underscored are the problematic relations of the fieldwork process which can become fluid, unstable, and contested, especially for feminist geographers when patriarchy is at stake.[40] In such male-dominated contexts, feminist researchers are forcefully "inserted in the grid of power relations."[41] Nonetheless, these power laden and socially fraught relations are often problematized with respect to researcher-subject relationships, and not subject-researcher relations.

Although I was unprepared for this patriarchal encounter, it expanded the boundaries of how I imagined subject-researcher relations, in particular, the ways that research subjects can wield untold power in the field. It also heightened my sense of positionality with regard to my power and privilege relative to the local HIV women. This is in the sense that as a woman in the field conducting feminist research, I was in some ways subject to these same constricting patriarchal forces that were so poignantly captured in the testimonials of the HIV-seropositive women. Yet there were other axes of my identity, for example, my social and class locations that provided me agency to negotiate how much these forces could regulate me.

Within the theory and practice of gender (and development) research, these field encounters bear multiple implications. Foremost, they essentialize how feminist researchers are confronted with the difficult task of navigating and negotiating the fine lines around the push for gender equality in steeply patriarchal societies given our identities as women, and the ways that this interacts with patriarchy to unintentionally shape our feminist agenda. Second, they reify a highly contested paradox which is the notion that female activism is deeply intertwined with cultural and gender politics, which may serve to reproduce injustices against women because in the attempts to address patriarchy, male dominance may be reproduced and reinforced as female activists get entangled in the very structures that they try to resist. Intertwined with this argument is also the role of class and social locations of feminist actors as they may unintentionally reproduce a nonrepresentational politics such that their activism addresses their own needs and interests—a subject that I discuss extensively in chapter 5 of this book. Third, these experiences insinuate that the concept of gender equality in Nigeria may have gained wider acceptance and reception over time because it has become both a global and a local policy fad that institutional stakeholders identify with for relevance but it is devoid of instrumentality. In practice, the concept of gender equality remains a threat to men and, sometimes, women too. As such, it continues to attract resistance from both the political elites and the grassroots, especially when the phrase is used in women-specific contexts or in ways that exclude male interests. Gender equality in development circles may thus have assumed a form of tokenism because while this branded term may be deployed increasingly, its true import has not been significantly grasped.[42] I build on this argument in the next paragraphs.

Nalia Kabeer's argument on the role of cultural power and politics as significant to the ways that gender mainstreaming is practiced in development institutions also speaks directly to the agenda of gender equality in patriarchal contexts where mainstream national policies may reflect the existing social order and determine how meanings around gender become constituted in ways that may be disconnected from the realities and psychosocial needs of women.[43] A classic example of this is the problematic abstraction of gender in very neutral ways, whether in pure universalistic and West-centric notions that occlude local understandings, devoid of any specificity to place and context, and thereby, produce ineffectual gender outcomes with no change to the existing social *status quo*.[44] Such problematic constructions effectuate the need for gender deconstruction in ways that provide insights into its "structural, ideological . . . and cultural entrapments," as well as other associated constraints within the relations of masculinities and femininities.[45]

Critical arguments are, therefore, made in this book for the use of intersectional and relational gender frameworks as well as the need to advance the notion that theorizations of gender must recognize the social dynamics and agencies of both male and female bodies, and see them as intricately intertwined.[46] In feminist studies, the theories of relationality and intersectionality speak directly to the platform on which transformative and innovative health policies must be circumscribed because these frameworks embody great possibilities for creating an effective understanding of gender issues.[47] This, in turn, demands an understanding of the varied conceptualizations of gender and their implication for policy and development actions in health interventions.

Nongovernmental Organizations

Another issue at stake that is also vital to the discourse on the barriers to effective gender mainstreaming that this book illuminates is the role of institutional power relations at the national and transnational levels. Across these scales, there are the not-so-visible institutional forces, for example, the machinery of transnational governance through donor funding relationships that reperpetuate institutional bottlenecks around the effective incorporation of gender into treatment interventions on the local landscape.

The immanent and intentional development activities of international governance systems, the global political economy, and transnational networks of aid through the NGO mechanism and bilateral and multilateral arrangements constitute a complex arrangement that regulates and complicates the ways that global health interventions are localized and implemented.[48] NGOs have been argued to be indirect tools for global-local policy transfer through their connections to transnational funding networks which not only drive their local agenda but also structure and condition the forms of knowledge integrated into local interventions.[49] The unequal power relationship between international donor funding bodies and NGOs undermines the generic capabilities of these grassroots organizations to streamline local context into development strategies in locally appropriate ways.

The role of NGOs in critical development studies has garnered increasing attention by critical human geographers and development scholars in contemporary research and for good reasons.[50] Given the failures of mainstream economic development policies, the NGO landscape emerged as a viable space and mechanism for *alternative* development practices that engender genuine social and transformative change because of NGOs perceived comparative advantage with local populations and place-based knowledge.[51] NGOs have, thus, continued to assume significance within the alternative development paradigm. As part of civil society and non-state actors, NGOs are largely perceived to be capable of producing more empowering and sustainable forms of development through grounded local knowledges of people and places, in dissonance with the exclusionary practices of mainstream development.[52] Also significant is that their non-state nature and affiliations with local geographies and grassroots organizations position them to act as counter social movements to mainstream national development projects, with the ability to rework traditional meanings of interventions in ways that are socially, culturally, and politically meaningful, as well as empowering to local populations.[53]

Over time, the increasing professionalization of many NGOs, emanating from their dualized nature with simultaneously constitutive relations to transnational forces of aid, the state, and neoliberal market, on the one hand, and local interests, on the other, has cast doubts on the propensity of NGOs to be an alternative development machine.[54] This growing doubt has produced a schism in development theory and practice between those who laud NGOs as the "institutional alternative to existing development" practices and critical skeptics who call for more caution about the ability of NGOs to implement a development agenda different from the official norm, given their connections to colonial actors, with the argument that NGOs could be indirect agents of neo-imperialism.[55] Some skeptics even argue that NGOs have increasingly become the Trojan horses of global neoliberalism.[56] Hence, development scholars have called for the need to develop a recognition and awareness of the politics of the so-called NGO development expertise manifesting through alliances with non-state transnational actors as they foster new but intricate and complex practices of development.[57] For example, there is evidence that the uneven spatialization of NGOs is serving to "pluralize particular spaces and places at the expense of others."[58] This is in addition to the growing concern that NGOs are now intricately tied to the very neoliberal agenda that they were designed to critically engage, as alternative actors to mainstream development.[59]

Such agitations have also produced calls for NGOs to be conceptualized as they actually exist in their true forms, that is, as units subsumed within this larger web of global institutions and translocal forces but not as neutral organizations with distinct boundaries that are divorced from their parent institutions.[60] The typical but erroneously assumed separation of NGOs from their transnational structure produces a less objective analysis of NGOs. Nonetheless, the task of fully deconstructing the complex connections that NGOs make with their parent institutions is beyond the scope of this book but the analysis does well to circumscribe the practices of local NGOs responsible for HIV treatment in Nigeria, as well as their trajectories of interventions, within these transnational tendencies and global funding relations.

The propensity for NGOs to become effective tools for civil society change and transformation is not in debate or in doubt but what is controversial and also highly contested is their capability to do so because of their alliances with the broader systems of global policy governance. This is a recurrent premise throughout the alternative and critical development literature. It is also one that has shaped the perspective this book takes on the subject of the NGO machinery and the ways that this may reproduce uneven development and gendered inequalities. A key assumption made here is that the transnational tendencies of NGOs may work through specific languages and technologies to produce the exclusion of certain local priorities and also (re)marginalize particular groups. Within this discourse, this book provides clarity on specific ways that NGO complexities reproduce uneven development and inequalities for women in developing world spaces.

Needs- and Rights-Based Discourses

Also significant to the dialogue on en*gendering* transformative development is the debate between needs- and rights-based approaches as effective strategies for incorporating women into development policies.[61] In a study of development discourses in Africa, Ben Wisner showcased the relevance of a *needs-rights*-based model and advocated for this dual approach to development.[62] However, in more recent development studies, arguments have been mostly made for a rights-based approach to incorporate women into the development map.[63] Following Wisner, I argue that the needs- and the rights-based approaches should not be considered as mutually exclusive but as a dual approach that can produce a strong synergy when deployed collaboratively to mainstream women into development.

In my analysis, I acknowledge the inherent limitations of the needs- and the rights-based approaches. Also intrinsic to this argument is how local cultures and traditional practices can shape not only the ways needs are articulated and by whom but also the problematic ways that rights are invoked and claimed by less dominant and marginalized groups of women in patriarchal societies. Also paramount is a necessity to elucidate indigenous practices of rights as they are entangled with power and harmful gender ideologies in such spaces.[64]

Like rights, certain questions also have to be addressed around needs—who should define needs, should it be the poor people or development experts or intervention agencies; what does satisfying a need entail, would it be "simply to deliver packages of 'needs meeting' services (water pumps, health care, emergency bags of grain) as aid agencies so often do, or must poor people control the resources required to meet their needs?"[65] In spite of the inherent limitations of these approaches, there is an argument that can be made for both in the absence or lack of more effective alternatives, and I highlight some of these gains and how they can be leveraged upon to further advance women in development thought and practice.

Still, I provide a cautionary tale that the intrinsic values of a needs-rights-based strategy should not be taken *prima facie* or as devoid of problems, especially when practiced within specific spatial contexts. In this book, I clarify the specific ways I recommend this combined approach as a solution for a more participatory gender framework. Within the context of the Niger Delta region—patriarchy, resource marginalization, and struggle for the rights to determine and control resources—a needs-right-based approach is significant for local knowledge especially around the ways that the needs and rights of poor women can become further subverted. Or alternatively, the effective ways women's needs and rights can be inserted into the development agenda.

All of these essential debates profoundly shape the ways that this book interrogates the role of development institutions, gender, and cultural power in HIV treatment access and adherence with the argument that these factors are immensely crucial to how we can understand the health-seeking behaviors of HIV-seropositive women. The analysis of the role of institutional power as a determinant of gendered health access and adherence also presents a finely honed sensitivity to the failures of policy makers who talk about gender mainstreaming but fail to deliver real, sustainable health services for disenfranchised women suffering from the social stigma and alienation associated with HIV seropositivity.

The perspectives offered in this book provide important policy and programmatic insights into what are (non)effective HIV treatment interventions for relevant governments, bilateral and multilateral organizations, as well as international NGOs (INGOs), and also with an aim to narrow the divide between development theory and practice. This does not in any way preclude the fact that sometimes there are impracticalities in proactively translating the critique of social and public health policies into effective action. In the least, what is aimed for is that the lived experiences and realities of women living with HIV will continue to foster local-global conversations and (re)configure existing practices, in order to create effective linkages between HIV/AIDS science and public social policies in developing world contexts.

ABOUT THE BOOK

Pathologies of Patriarchy: Death, Suffering, Care, and Coping in the Gendered Gaps of HIV/AIDS Interventions in Nigeria offers readers a window into a world of suffering, coping, and care especially at a time when access to ARV drugs has become widespread in West Africa. Yet significant gaps in access, adherence to treatment, and retention in care remain.[66]

With 1.9 million people living with HIV/AIDS as of 2018, Nigeria has the largest HIV/AIDS epidemic in West Africa.[67] Despite the fact that the country's HIV/AIDS prevalence rate declined from 3.2 percent in 2016 to 1.9 percent in 2018, a 2019 UNAIDS report states that Nigeria, along with Cameroon and Côte d'Ivoire, account for about 60 percent of new HIV infections and 54 percent of AIDS-related deaths in West Africa annually. Hence, significant improvements in these countries national HIV programs would wield a major positive impact on the region's HIV response. Nigeria also lags behind many West African countries in ART coverage.[68] Even among those receiving ART therapy in the region, knowledge and data on retention rates remain scarce but with retention in care generally estimated to be suboptimal.[69] According to a UNAIDS 2016 report, an even greater need lies in uncovering treatment and retention gaps at the national level because "the trend towards increased ARV therapy coverage across Africa masks significant national gaps."[70] The extremely limited national- and region-specific information on the subject necessitates a dire need to situate the site of this research in Nigeria. This book addresses this knowledge gap not only within the scholarship of HIV/AIDS but also within the domain of policy.

The essentialization of the HIV/AIDS epidemic using particular geographies in sub-Saharan Africa is a common feature in most HIV/AIDS discourses. As such, very little is known about this epidemic in other parts of the continent because knowledge of particular regions in the east and the south that have been well studied is used to popularize existing discourses.[71] Such reductionist analyses limit our understanding of the geography of HIV treatment in sub-Saharan Africa. Through the lens of Nigeria, this book draws scholarly attention to the HIV treatment discourse in one of the less studied regions of the continent, West Africa.[72] While the lessons about the barriers women face when seeking HIV treatment from existing analyses on South and East Africa are also germane to other parts of the continent, it is important to have a robust scholarship on the sub-Saharan African HIV treatment discourse.

Central to the design of this book, therefore, is its ability to make this sort of almost contradictory juxtaposition in that it takes both a specific and a generalist approach to understand the issues. This book situates the HIV treatment discourse within a particular spatial context while it simultaneously draws compelling insights from other national contexts in sub-Saharan Africa. As well as being inter-regionally relevant, the arguments made in this book are of great disciplinary and interdisciplinary interests to a wide variety of scholars, whether they are researching gendered inequality from a geographical, anthropological, or global health lens or are interested in broader concerns about development and inequality in sub-Saharan Africa. HIV/AIDS researchers, students, policy makers, development practitioners, and anyone interested in HIV/AIDS in sub-Saharan Africa are able to fully comprehend the issues in the way that this book brings together the experiential analysis of the personal and body politics to the local and global within a single analytical framework.

Using critical discourse analysis, observations, focus group discussions, and in-depth interviews conducted among HIV-seropositive women and national policy stakeholders, the analysis made in this book has emerged from a qualitative research inquiry conducted in one of Nigeria's most complex geographies, the Niger Delta. By leveraging on ground evidence and real-time testimonials envisioned through the everyday lived realities of HIV-seropositive women in the Niger Delta region, the associated complexities of this region also provide a unique perspective to understand the web of factors that underpin women's health-seeking behavior in complicated geographies, especially where patriarchy is at force.

The uniqueness of this book's design also lies in the way it brings together a feminist geographical analysis of gendered inequalities around HIV treatment with practical implementation questions concerning the limits of current global health programming using a multiscalar lens such that we do not only benefit from hearing the voices of the women most impacted but also simultaneously engage the views of those at the perimeter of power and change. Such a linkage provides both theoretical and practical pathways for understanding women's personal struggles with treatment through a personal and structural lens.

While I do not entertain utopian thoughts or ambitions that this book will or can erase all inequalities around treatment among HIV-seropositive women, the goal is to expose the unequal conditions that consume their daily lives and how these may create risky but avoidable vulnerabilities in the domain of treatment, and consequently, unhealthy outcomes. Similarly, the aim is to draw conscious attention to these social inequities in the hope that they can be at least addressed through institutionalized policy instruments that effectively mainstream women's social realities. It is hoped that through such interpretive discourses which reflect grassroots experiences using the lens of HIV-seropositive women and the perspectives of policy makers, this book will help to unseat the hegemonic biomedical discourses on HIV/AIDS and improve seemingly well-intentioned intervention models that prioritize the technical aspects of ARVs over the social realities that produce inequities in access, adherence, and retention in care.

I also make a disclaimer that the depth of analysis of the relevant scholarships on related topics throughout this book represents the full scope and extent of these scholarships. From the inception of this work, my aim was to represent as much as it is possible the voices of the HIV-seropositive women I worked with, as well as the policy stakeholders. If I did not fully delve into particular dimensions of the scholarships referenced in this book, it is because these do not directly or indirectly speak to the range of data that emerged from this work. But it is my utmost hope that this book does justice to the voices of the HIV-seropositive women who gave me the honor and pleasure of entering into their lives of seropositivity.

ORGANIZATION OF THE BOOK

The remaining chapters in this book are organized into three parts: history, politics, and HIV/AIDS governance; embodied accounts; and models of interventions.

Part 1: "History, Politics, and HIV/AIDS Governance" situate the context in which to understand broadly, the geography of HIV/AIDS in Nigeria. Chapter 2 provides a historical perspective on the emergence of the HIV/AIDS epidemic; a broad overview of the epidemic; and the concomitant social, political, and policy response through different timelines and political eras in Nigeria. Subsequent analysis in chapter 3 narrows this discourse to provide a regional perspective. This chapter unpacks the intersection of social, gender, and political power with the investments of transnational oil corporations in the Niger Delta region, as they pattern ARV access and produce a unique geography of HIV care among women.

Part 2: "Embodied Accounts" illuminate the multidimensional nature of ARV access and adherence by unpacking the roles of traditional cultural systems and health systems governance as they structure women's decision-making in seeking treatment and negotiating the barriers to care. This part begins with chapter 4, which addresses a key theoretical debate in the feminist care ethics scholarship, the notions of care and responsibility as experienced within patriarchal relations and social contexts. Chapter 5 examines the plethora of ways that women rationalize the decision to disclose or not, the ways that disclosure by women disrupts intimate relations, for example, spousal abandonment, and how this is fast reconfiguring the structure of the traditional family unit with the increasing number of female-headed households. Chapter 6 explores the issues of representational politics and feminist activism on gender equality in Nigeria, and how the equality agenda is understood and pursued by feminist activists whose class and social locations shape in significantly profound ways, the polarizing discourses of empowerment between local women and elite feminist actors. Chapter 7 is an in-depth examination of HIV/AIDS support groups as the most critical coping outlet for HIV-seropositive women to negotiate the barriers to access and adherence to treatment. The chapter presents a detailed analysis of the ways that HIV/AIDS support networks as biomedical safety nets are constantly being reconfigured to become micro-therapeutic spaces, and sites for the accumulation of social and economic capital within the formal healthcare landscape. Perceptions of HIV/AIDS interventions especially as they parallel the divide between the biomedical and the biosocial aspects of treatment are also discussed. Besides these support networks are other strategies that HIV-seropositive women deploy to negotiate and cope with the constraints to treatment. These are explored in chapter 8. Also significant to this discourse is the increasing connection between faith-based practices and coping with HIV/AIDS. Chapter 8 links weak institutional responsibility and the culture of individualized health responsibility as significant to the choices women make to cope. It illuminates how women's narrative accounts mirror current debates on the exceptionalism and normalization of HIV/AIDS.

In Part 3: "Models of Interventions," chapter 9 presents a detailed examination of the concept of gender mainstreaming. It exposes the barriers to effective gender mainstreaming practice in development work and problematizes these within the context of institutional (local and transnational) power relations. Chapter 10 takes a critical look at existing models and approaches to gender mainstreaming within a health and development framework. It is also the conclusion about a work that is unending because action starts where this book ends. In this final chapter, I also reconcile the debates and arguments made in the preceding chapters as well as their implications for biomedical interventions in arenas that have been shown to be predominantly influenced by social forces.

NOTES

1. Gita Ramjee and Brodie Daniels, "Women and HIV in Sub-Saharan Africa," *AIDS Research and Therapy* 10, no. 30 (December 2013): 5–6, https://doi.org/10.1186/1742-6405-10-30.

2. See Ippolytos A. Kalofonos, "'All I Eat Is ARVs': The Paradox of AIDS Treatment Interventions in Central Mozambique," *Medical Anthropology Quarterly* 24, no. 3 (2010): 363–380, https://doi.org/10.1111/j.1548–1387.2010.01109.x.

3. WLWHA stands for Women Living with HIV/AIDS but in the context of this book, I use Women Living with HIV (WLWH) because in the practice of ARTs, treatment at the diseased stage of the virus (AIDS) is usually not initiated because it is considered ineffective. The focus is therefore, on women who are at the infectious stage of the virus and eligible for treatment based on CD4 500 cells/mm^3 or less as standard practice.

4. Paul E. Farmer et al., "Structural Violence and Clinical Medicine," *PLoS Medicine* 3, no. 10 (October 2006): 1686, https://doi.org/10.1371/journal.pmed.0030449; Paul Farmer, *Infections and Inequalities: The Modern Plagues* (Berkeley: University of California Press, 1999), 79.

5. Farmer, *Infections and Inequalities*, 79, 85.

6. Susan Craddock, "Beyond Epidemiology: Locating AIDS in Africa," in *HIV and AIDS in Africa: Beyond Epidemiology*, eds. Ezekiel Kalipeni, Susan Craddock, Joseph R. Oppong, and Jayati Ghosh (Oxford: Blackwell, 2004), 4–5.

7. Caroline Faria, "Privileging Prevention, Gender Responsibility: An Analysis of the Ghanaian Campaign against AIDS," *Social and Cultural Geography* 9, no. 1 (February 2008): 42, https://doi.org/10.1080/14649360701789584.

8. Michael Kevane, *Women and Development in Africa: How Gender Works* (Boulder, CO: Lynne Rienner, 2004), 1.

9. See Ramjee and Daniels, "Women and HIV in Sub-Saharan Africa."

10. Alison Mountz and Jennifer Hyndman, "Feminist Approaches to the Global Intimate," *Women's Studies Quarterly* 34, no. 1/2 (Spring 2006): 446; Farmer, *Infections and Inequalities*, 258–259.

11. United Nations, *The World's Women 2015: Trends and Statistics* (New York: United Nations Department of Economic and Social Affairs, 2015), 13, https://unstats.un.org/unsd/gender/downloads/worldswomen2015_report.pdf.

12. See Mark Hunter, *Love in the Time of AIDS: Inequality, Gender and Rights in South Africa* (Bloomington: Indiana University Press, 2010).

13. See Faria, "Privileging Prevention, Gender Responsibility"; Hunter, *Love in the Time of AIDS*; and Farmer's works as hitherto cited.

14. Robin Kearns and Damian Collins, "Health Geography," in *A Companion to Health and Medical Geography*, eds. Tim Brown, Sara McLafferty, and Graham Moon (Oxford: Wiley-Blackwell, 2010), 16–17. Also see Robin Kearns and Graham Moon, "From Medical to Health Geography: Novelty, Place and Theory after a Decade of Change," *Progress in Human Geography* 26, no. 5 (2002), https://doi.org/10.1191/0309132502ph389oa.

15. Vani S. Kulkarni and Subu V. Subramanian, "Social Perspectives on Health Inequalities," in *A Companion to Health and Medical Deography*, eds. Tim Brown, Sara McLafferty, and Graham Moon (Oxford: Wiley-Blackwell, 2010), 378.

16. Erhoike community which houses the healthcare facility where HIV-seropositive women investigated accessed HIV treatment is the actual site of study. For detailed description, see chapter 3.

17. Raymond L. Bryant, "Political Ecology: An Emerging Research Agenda in Third World Studies," *Political Geography* 11, no. 1 (January 1992): 14–15. Also see People's Health Movement, Medact and Global Equity Gauge Alliance, *Global Health Watch 2: An Alternative World Health Report* (London: Zed Books, 2008).

18. Donna Haraway, "Situated Knowledges: The Science Question in Feminism and the Privilege of Partial Perspective," *Feminist Studies* 14, no. 3 (Fall 1988): 590.

19. Susan Craddock, "Disease, Social Identity and Risk: Rethinking the Geography of AIDS," *Transactions of the Institute of British Geographers* 25, no. 2 (2000): 164–165.

20. Melissa W. Wright, "Geography and Gender: Feminism and a Feeling of Justice," *Progress in Human Geography* 34, no. 6 (2010): 821, https://doi.org/10.1177/0309132510362931.

21. Kalofonos, "'All I Eat Is ARVs'," 364.

22. Alan Greig et al., "Gender and AIDS: Time to Act," *AIDS* 22, no. 2 (August 2008): 2, https://doi.org/10.1097/01.aids.0000327435.28538.18.

23. Janet Seeley, Rachel Grellier, and Tony Barnett, "Gender and HIV/AIDS Impact Mitigation in Sub-Saharan Africa: Recognizing the Constraints," *Journal of Social Aspects of HIV/AIDS* 1, no. 2 (August 2004): 94.

24. "Nigeria Opens 41 New AIDS Treatment Centers," *Reuters*, last modified March 14, 2006, http://www.aegis.org/news/re/2006/RE060316.html.

25. National Agency for the Control of AIDS, *National HIV/AIDS Strategic Plan 2010–2015* (Abuja: National Agency for the Control of AIDS, 2009), 18.

26. National Agency for the Control of AIDS, *Global AIDS Response: Country Progress Report, Nigeria* (Abuja: National Agency for the Control of AIDS, 2015), ix, http://www.unaids.org/sites/default/files/country/documents/NGA_narrative_report_2015.pdf.

27. United Nations, *Nigeria - United Nations Sustainable Development Partnership Framework (UNSDPF) 2018 to 2022* (Abuja: United Nations, 2017), 13, http://www.ng.undp.org/content/nigeria/en/home/library/knowledgeproducts/un-sustainable-development-partnership-framework-2018-2022.html; National Agency for the Control of AIDS, *HIV/AIDS National Strategic Framework for Action 2005–2009* (Abuja: Society for Family Health, 2005), 20.

28. "Nigeria: Progress towards 90-90-90 Target," UNAIDS, accessed July 31, 2019, http://aidsinfo.unaids.org/.

29. João Biehl, "When People Come First: Beyond Technical and Theoretical Quick-Fixes in Global Health," in *Global Political Ecology*, eds. Richard Peet, Paul Robbins, and Michael J. Watts (London: Routledge, 2011), 111–112; Kalofonos, " 'All I Eat Is ARVs'," 363.

30. Bernhard Schwartländer, Ian Grubb, and Jos Perriëns, "The 10-Year Struggle to Provide Antiretroviral Treatment to People with HIV in the Developing World," *Lancet* 368 (August 2006): 544; Biehl, "When People Come First," 102; Also see Tina Rosenberg, "Look at Brazil," *New York Times*, January 28, 2001; Kalofonos, " 'All I Eat Is ARVs'."

31. Thomas C. Ricketts, "Accessing Health Care," in *A Companion to Health and Medical Geography*, eds. Tim Brown, Sara McLafferty, and Graham Moon (Oxford: Wiley-Blackwell, 2010), 522.

32. For example, see Ricketts, "Accessing Health Care," 522–523; Policy Brief, *Access Challenges for HIV Treatment among People Living with HIV and Key Populations in Middle-Income Countries* (2013), https://msmgf.org/wp-content/uploads/2015/09/Access_Challenges_for_HIV_treatment_KAPs.pdf.

33. World Health Organization, *Consolidated Guidelines on the Use of Antiretroviral Drugs for Treating and Preventing HIV Infection* (Geneva: WHO, 2013), 176, https://www.who.int/hiv/pub/guidelines/arv2013/operational/en/.

34. Ibid., 176.

35. See Ayalu A. Reda and Sibhatu Biadgilign, "Determinants of Adherence to Antiretroviral Therapy among HIV-Infected Patients in Africa," *AIDS Research and Treatment* 2012 (February 2012): 1–8, https:// doi.org/10.1155/2012/574656; Elvin Geng, "Retention in Care for HIV-Infected Patients in Resource-Limited Settings: Challenges and Opportunities," *HIV InSite*, last modified January 2011, http://hivinsite.ucsf.edu/InSite?page=md-expert-geng.

36. World Health Organization, *Consolidated Guidelines*, 176.

37. Geng, "Retention in Care."

38. Ibid.

39. Paul Farmer, *AIDS and Accusation: Haiti and the Geography of Blame* (Berkeley: University of California, 1992), 247–249.

40. See Emily Billo and Nancy Hiemstra, "Mediating Messiness: Expanding Ideas of Flexibility, Reflexivity, and Embodiment in Fieldwork," *Gender, Place and Culture: A Journal of Feminist Geography* 20, no. 3 (2013), https://doi.org/10.1080/0966369X.2012.674929.

41. José Medina, *Speaking from Elsewhere: A New Contextualist Perspective Meaning, Identity and Discursive Agency* (Albany: State University of New York Press, 2006), 126.

42. Sylvia H. Chant and Cathy McIlwaine, *Geographies of Development in the 21st Century: An Introduction to the Global South* (Cheltenham, UK: Edward Edgar, 2003), 223.

43. Nalia Kabeer, *Reversed Realities: Gender, Hierarchies in Development Thought* (London: Verso, 1994), 35–36, 269.

44. Raewyn Connell, "Gender, Health and Theory: Conceptualizating the Issue in Local and World Perspective," *Social Science and Medicine* 74 (2012): 1680, https://doi.org/ 10.1016/j.socscimed.2011.06.006; Kabeer, *Reversed Realities*, 269.

45. Also see Anne Akeroyd, "Coercion, Constraints and 'Cultural Entrapments': A Further Look at Gendered and Occupational Factors Pertinent to the Transmission of HIV in Africa," in *HIV and AIDS in Africa: Beyond Epidemiology*, eds. Ezekiel Kalipeni, Susan Craddock, Joseph R. Oppong, and Jayati Ghosh (Oxford: Blackwell, 2004), 101; Hunter, *Love in the Time of AIDS*, 11.

46. Connell, "Gender, Health and Theory," 1678.

47. Ibid., 1677. Also see Olena Hankvisky, "Women's Health, Men's Health and Gender and Health: Implications of Intersectionality," *Social Science and Medicine* 74 (2012), https://doi.org/10.1016/j.socscimed.2011.11.029; Kristen W. Springer, Olena Hankivsky, and Lisa M. Bates, "Gender and Health: Relational, Intersectional, and Biosocial Approaches," *Social Science and Medicine* 74, no. 11 (March 2012), https://doi.org/ 10.1016/j.socscimed.2012.03.001; Kristen W. Springer, Jeanne M. Stellman, and Rebecca M. Jordan-Young, "Beyond a Catalogue of Differences: A Theoretical Frame and Good Practice Guidelines for Researching Sex/Gender in Human Health," *Social Science and Medicine* 74 (2012), https://doi.org/10.1016/j.socscimed.2011.05.033.

48. See Richa Nagar and Saraswati Raju, "Women, NGOs, and the Contradictions of Empowerment and Disempowerment: A Conversation," *Antipode* 35, no. 1 (February 2003), https://doi.org/10.1111/1467-8330.00298; For meanings of development as an immanent or unintentional process, and as an intentional activity, see Diana Mitlin, Sam Hickey, and Anthony Bebbington, "Reclaiming Development? NGOs and the Challenge of Alternatives," *World Development* 35, no. 10 (2007): 1701, https:// doi.org/10.1016/j.worlddev.2006.11.005. Also see Anthony Bebbington, "NGOs and Uneven Development: Geographies of Development Intervention," *Progress in Human Geography* 28, no. 6 (2004): 725–726, https://doi.org/10.1191/0309132504ph516oa.

49. Hakan Seckinelgin, "A Global Disease and Its Governance: HIV/AIDS in Sub-Saharan Africa and the Agency of NGOs," *Global Governance* 11, no. 3 (2005): 357–358.

50. For example, see Matthew Sparke, "Health," in *The SAGE Handbook of Progress in Human Geography*, eds. Roger Lee, Noel Castree, Rob Kitchin, Vicky Lawson, Anssi Paasi, Sarah Radcliffe, and Charles Withers (Thousand Oaks, CA: Sage, 2014). Also see Bebbington, "NGOs and Uneven Development," 727.

51. Mitlin, Hickey, and Bebbington, "Reclaiming Development," 1701.

52. Ibid.

53. Anne Gordon Drabek, "Development Alternatives: The Challenge for NGOs - an Overview of the Issues," *World Development* 15 (1987): x, xiii. Also see Arturo Escobar, "Histories of Development, Predicaments of Modernity: Thinking about Globalization from Some Critical Development Studies Perspective," in *Rural Transformation and Development - China in Context: The Everyday Lives of Policies*

and People, eds. Norman Long, Ye Jingzhong, and Wang Yihuan (Cheltenham, UK: Edward Elgar, 2010), 29–33.

54. Nagar and Raju, "Women, NGOs, and the Contradictions of Empowerment and Disempowerment," 12.

55. Mitlin, Hickey, and Bebbington, "Reclaiming Development," 1700; Bebbington, "NGOs and Uneven Development," 728.

56. Arundhati Roy, "The NGO-ization of Resistance," *Toward Freedom*, last modified September 8, 2014, http://www.towardfreedom.com/33-archives/globalism/3660-arundhati-roy-the-ngo-ization-of-resistance. Also see David Harvey, *A Brief History of Neoliberalism* (New York: Oxford University Press, 2005).

57. See Escobar, "Histories of Development, Predicaments of Modernity," 33.

58. Claire Mercer, "NGOs, Civil Society and Democratization: A Critical Review of the Literature," *Progress in Development Studies* 2, no.1 (2002): 13, https://doi.org/10.1191/1464993402ps027ra; Bebbington, "NGOs and Uneven Development," 740–741.

59. Mitlin, Hickey, and Bebbington, "Reclaiming Development," 1706.

60. Bebbington, "NGOs and Uneven Development," 728–729.

61. Cathy Mcllwaine and Kavita Data, "From Feminizing to Engendering Development," *Gender, Place and Culture* 10, no. 4 (2003): 371, 373, https://doi.org/10.1080/0966369032000155564. Also see Hunter, *Love in the Time of AIDS*, 9.

62. Ben Wisner. *Power and Need in Africa* (Trenton: Africa World Press, 1982).

63. See, for example, Greig et al., "Gender and AIDS," 3, 5.

64. Mcllwaine and Datta, "From Feminizing to Engendering Development," 374.

65. Wisner, *Power and Need in Africa*, 13.

66. Medecins Sans Frontiers, *Out of Focus: How Millions of People in West and Central Africa Are Being Left Out of the Global HIV Response* (Medecins Sans Frontiers, 2016), 10–13, https://www.msf.org/sites/msf.org/files/2016_04_hiv_report_eng.pdf.

67. "AIDS Info: Nigeria," UNAIDS, accessed August 8, 2019, http://aidsinfo.unaids.org/.

68. "AIDS Info"; UNAIDS, *UNAIDS Data 2019* (Geneva: UNAIDS, 2019), 76, https://www.unaids.org/sites/default/files/media_asset/2019-UNAIDS-data_en.pdf. Also see Medecins Sans Frontiers, *Out of Focus*, 10.

69. Plazy et al., "Retention in Care Prior to Antiretroviral Treatment Eligibility in Sub-Saharan Africa: A Systematic Review of the Literature," *BMJ Open* 5 (2015): 8, https://doi.org/10.1136/bmjopen-2014–006927; Medecins Sans Frontiers, *Out of Focus*, 11.

70. UNAIDS, *Access to Antiretroviral Therapy in Africa: Status Report on Progress towards the 2015 Targets* (UNAIDS, 2013), 4, http://www.unaids.org/sites/default/files/media_asset/20131219_AccessARTAfricaStatusReportProgresstowards2015Targets_en_0.pdf.

71. See Plazy et al., "Retention in Care Prior to Antiretroviral Treatment Eligibility in Sub-Saharan Africa," 8.

72. Medecins Sans Frontiers, *Out of Focus*, 4.

Chapter 2

HIV/AIDS in Nigeria: Denialism and Response

In this chapter, I detail the emergence of the HIV/AIDS epidemic in Nigeria and the concomitant policy response from historical and gender perspectives, and how these have shaped the current landscape of intervention. I problematize the emergence, response, and features of the Nigerian HIV/AIDS epidemic within the broader sub-Saharan African HIV/AIDS discourse as these are intricately intertwined.

The first two cases of AIDS in Nigeria were discovered in 1985, during the era of military dictatorship and political instability but reported to the Federal Ministry of Health (FMoH) in 1986.[1] Like many sub-Saharan African countries, Nigeria's response was emblematic of the global HIV/AIDS political climate in the early stage of the pandemic. Nigeria responded to this disease with disbelief and tagged it as the figment of scientists' imagination.[2] At the time, knowledge about the geographical origin of the virus was very much contested and most of the African origin theses that were perpetuated were regarded as myths, especially by African scholars because of the racial undertones and the lack of definite scientific evidence.[3] Contradictory evidence surrounding the African evolution theory further fueled the controversy, producing a divide among scholars whereby most Western literature argued in favor of an African origin theory, while non-Western scholars refuted this claim.[4] Western conceptualizations of AIDS in Africa as emergent of barbaric African customs were also well hyped by the American media.[5] African scholars argued that such constructions emanated from misconstrued colonial and neocolonial understandings of the African culture, as well as metaphorical constructions of Africa as a Dark Continent.[6] African governments and researchers thus rejected this cultural theory and met the notion of an African AIDS epidemic with skepticism, disapproval, and resistance. In Nigeria, HIV/AIDS metamorphosed into a major public health issue, in part, due to these prevailing perceptions. The poor reception that greeted its discovery in the continent also led to a delayed response and inaction by the government, and these were exacerbated by a lack of political will. The unaddressed epidemiological drivers of the disease largely from heterosexual transmission, blood transfusion, presence of sexually transmitted infections (STIs), mother-to-child transmission, stigmatization and discrimination, as well as harmful sociocultural norms and practices also intensified the epidemic.[7]

Like many African nations, the Nigerian HIV/AIDS epidemic can also be argued to have emerged and escalated from a broad spectrum of social, political, and economic complexities ranging from corruption, legacies of colonialism, and racism that weakened nations' character, and from global political-economic processes like structural adjustment programs (SAPs) that not only contributed to the conditions that created spaces of high risks and vulnerabilities but also diminished available resources to curtail its spread.[8] In geographies like Nigeria, where women have a perceived lower social status in relation to men, a downswing in resources like the well-documented gendered impacts of SAPs could mean that women's already-controlled access to resources would further diminish.[9] In South Africa, the impact of global economic restructuring produced differential outcomes within and between gender groups with rich white males largely benefiting from the privatization of the industrial economic sector.[10] Similar to South Africa, Nigerian women in relation to men were, in general, more negatively impacted but there was a dual burden on poor, rural, and uneducated women.[11] Besides gender, therefore, income, education, and geographical location are other forms of social markers that shape inequalities for women—a reality that negates the erroneous assumption of women that is sometimes invoked in development policies and actions which is women as a monolithic and homogenous entity.

Recurrent statistics continue to depict the Nigerian HIV/AIDS epidemic as highly feminized with recent statistics indicating a 3.0 to 2.5 ratio of adult women aged fifteen to forty-nine years to men in the same category living with the virus; and 1.6 to 1.3 ratio of women to men in the fifteen years and above category.[12] This disparity in female-male prevalence rate may be reflexive of the pervasive gender inequalities that continue to characterize most heterosexual relationships engendered by fundamental patriarchal values. Not surprising, Nigeria ranked 118 out of 134 countries on the Gender Equality Index in 2016 because very little progress has been achieved in the promotion of gender equality.[13] Gender disparity in prevalence rates may also indicate that existing HIV/AIDS policies and programs may be failing to significantly lower this gap as unequal gender norms are inadvertently transferred to policy spaces—harmful norms that work to configure the so-called gender-sensitive policies which further reproduce gender gaps and widen the margins of risks and vulnerabilities for women. Patriarchal power at all levels of human activity may thus act to (in)directly empower certain socials groups and disadvantage or exclude others.

As a social system, patriarchy is almost synonymous with female oppression because its core principles celebrate male power and dominance at every scale of human activity and social relations. Patriarchal societies centralize a cultural, sociopolitical, and structural arrangement that legitimizes the social status of women mostly by their associations with men through marriage and kinship. Within patriarchal orders, women are mostly constructed as passive social and economic agents. Also, characteristic of this system is that unequal power allocation between the sexes translates to modes of resource control, distribution, access, and decision-making by men. The perceived notions of the naturalness of male superiority dominant in most African cultures thus underpin the social constructions and characterizations of gender in Nigeria, and other forms of inequalities that this book aims to destabilize.

HIV/AIDS in Nigeria, like most spaces in sub-Saharan Africa, is therefore about power—political power, gender power, and economic power whether by the state or individual.[14] Although biological factors may play a role (there is paucity of research providing strong evidence),[15] stark inequalities in gender relations continue to position females with a higher vulnerability risk index due to factors of subordination, discriminatory sociocultural practices, lack of control over sexual and reproductive decisions, material and financial dependence on men, intergenerational sex and marriages, and restrictions in control and access to resources that undermine the power of women to negotiate gender and social relations.[16]

Women's experiences of HIV/AIDS mirror the complex relationships between social and institutional structures, and the inequities associated with their gender especially at the household level where males define the terms of relations. Female subordination thus evolves from deeply entrenched traditional and religious values that institutionalize patriarchal norms and which objectify women and deem them inferior to men in all hierarchies of social and economic life. Nigeria's sociocultural milieu is such that women have little agency to control their lives and bodies, irrespective of age and marital status. To illustrate, most marital arrangements require women to seek their husband's consent before they can access health care or make crucial life decisions.[17] The practice of traditional bride payment by men in marital institutions also reifies the objectification of women because it legitimizes the misconception that women's bodies are the properties of men.[18] Religious beliefs and scripts also give agency to hegemonic masculinities and female heteronomy.

Nigeria operates a multifaceted constitution. The fundamental freedoms and human rights of every citizen are circumscribed within a constitution that is underpinned by common, statutory, and customary laws, as well as a religious legal system highly vested in patriarchal privilege. Nigeria's religious laws, which are intertwined with its customary legal system, also comprise Islamic Sharia laws which institutionalize violence against women through a variety of harmful regulations and practices, one of which is the legalization of underage marriage—a law that has come under intense scrutiny both locally and globally but with little counteraction. This law considers girls under eighteen years as marriageable and when married, to be considered legal adults, in contradiction to the statutory or common law that designates an adult to be an individual eighteen years and older.[19] Like Islam, biblical laws also objectify women.[20] Christianity operates on a fundamental principle of inequality between the sexes that privileges and empowers men but positions women as subordinates. Most Nigerian women have come to assume their identities within these normative and hegemonic socioreligious constructions, perceived as part of the divine natural order.[21]

Most postcolonial political cultures in patriarchal societies are male-dominated and so is the policy arena where unequal gender relations are reproduced.[22] Indeed, the organization, hierarchies, planning processes, and priorities of political and social institutions cannot be divested from the politics of resource ownership and control, as well as the everyday materialities of life and social relations in particular spaces.[23] As such, a deep-seated desire to preserve the natural order of things or an institutional defense of the existing social *status quo* by policy makers through traditional forms of knowledge is not uncommon.[24] Patriarchal values can thus be reenacted and reinforced through structures that (re)perpetuate economic dependence of women on men, female subservience, and discriminatory laws. In addition, some traditions and cultures within Nigeria prohibit the rights of women to access land, capital, and employment, as well as knowledge through formal education.[25]

Gender inequalities are, by implication, built into the organization of all traditional and institutional structures in Nigeria just as they are also immanent products of the existing social system. Inequalities in gender relations thus remain germane to the increasing HIV/AIDS prevalence among women in Nigeria, whether in their increasing vulnerabilities to and risk of the disease, or in the low premium and huge neglect of health services directed at their needs in both prevention efforts and support of those living with the virus/disease.[26] This further demonstrates that the performance of gender in real terms is not simple or abstract. Gender and how it is experienced in all spheres of human existence including health is contingent on these complex structural and social forces that must be engaged theoretically and practically in health research and interventions. This assertion segues into the next discourse—a historical-contemporary textual analysis of HIV/AIDS interventions in Nigeria, from inception to present with critical attention to the ideology, language, and constructions of gender, and related concepts as they frame the tone, nature, and direction of HIV/AIDS mitigation efforts.

The arguments and claims I present in the remainder of this chapter are based on a historical review and critical discourse analysis of HIV/AIDS policy documents and texts.[27] In it, I explore the ways that exclusionary gender interventions in Nigeria may have been created (or not) through highly abstract forms, meanings, and representations of gender, as well as hegemonic biomedical narratives that exclude the social aspects of health. The objective is to identify institutional gaps in past and existing HIV/AIDS policies as they frame the nation's gendered response to treatment. I also make a disclaimer that the empirical evidence presented here may not be wholly representative of all policy responses and actions on the epidemic but limited to the body of texts that were available to me and analyzed for the aforementioned stated objective. Caution should be deployed, therefore, to the generalizability of the evidence.

Following Michel Foucault's scholarship, I make the argument that a critical discourse analysis enables us to understand the invisible ways that HIV subjects become embedded in a web of politics and power relations. It does this by illuminating the specific ways that power is permeated through institutional processes using the constructions of languages and texts, in ways that oppress and disempower minority, powerless, and marginal groups.[28] Similarly, I engage the concept of discourse as intertextuality, that is, the interaction of texts that produce a coalition of languages and ideologies whose nuanced meanings may help to explain institutional barriers to women's unsustained access and adherence to HIV treatment and care.

A LANDSCAPE OF INTERVENTIONS

Since the first discovery of AIDS in Nigeria, the nation has undergone different phases of response to the epidemic. The panic that this discovery created within political circles prompted initial interventions like the National Expert Advisory Committee on AIDS (NEACA) that was set up through the nation's FMoH in 1986.[29] This was the nation's first programmatic response and it focused on detection and prevention. Shortly after, the National AIDS and STDs Control Program (NASCP) was established in 1988 to replace NEACA but it was still under the coordination of the FMoH.[30] Given the instability of the military regime at the time, little was done in this era to address the epidemic and programs were not as effective in curbing transmission rates, more so because there were many unknowns about the epidemic.

A period of hiatus ensued in the aftermath of NASCP until 1999, when the country transitioned into its first democratic regime, one that ushered in a more coordinated and active AIDS response through the establishment of the Presidential Commission on AIDS (PCA) and the National Action Committee on AIDS. Although NASCP still exists, it is strictly a health sector response with activities coordinated under the auspices of the FMoH. On the other hand, the National Action Committee on AIDS became a full-blown agency in 2007; currently, the National Agency for the Control of AIDS (NACA), which is the main coordinating body responsible for the nation's overall multisectoral response.[31] NACA is an independent commission that reports directly to the presidency.

It was from my interviews with policy stakeholders that I first learned about the chasm between NASCP and NACA whether in terms of planning, design, and implementation of HIV/AIDS policies or general coordination of efforts. This disconnect was recurrently pointed out but without any logical explanation or plausible reasons as to the existing *status quo*. In fact, some of the policy stakeholders declared the existence of these two ostensibly similar but parallel HIV/AIDS institutions as redundant. A redundancy that has created major gaps in the country's HIV/AIDS programming, given the duplication of efforts, and the appropriation of funds between the two bodies for HIV/AIDS programs. I use the word "ostensibly" because indeed, there are stark similarities in the functions that NASCP and NACA perform but as aforementioned, NACA is responsible for all the nation's related HIV/AIDS efforts while NASCP is limited to a sectoral response at the FMoH. Still, this does not negate the fact that the core agenda of both bodies, especially as it relates to HIV/AIDS mitigation activities broadly, appears to be equivalent.

As part of an emerging HIV/AIDS intervention landscape, Nigeria adopted a multisectoral approach as a response; in part, to the intersectional nature of the epidemic, and as a response to the "Three Ones" principle launched by the international HIV/AIDS community to promote a universal coordination in the fight against HIV/AIDS.[32] The "Three Ones" mandate the national response of developing countries to operate under one HIV/AIDS coordinating agency (in this case, NACA), one strategic plan (National Strategic Framework [NSF]), and one monitoring and evaluation system (MES).

A multisectoral response is a coalition of relevant public and private sector agencies with an aim to produce a multifaceted HIV/AIDS intervention that simultaneously targets multiple areas implicated in the epidemic such as gender and food security, among others. As with any syndicated enterprise, there have been significant challenges especially in terms of administration and coordination between and across relevant private and public sectors, ministries and parastatals, as well as the different tiers of program administration at the national, state, and local levels. An inherent challenge to this multisectoral approach has been the duplicity of efforts that has persisted from the early phase of interventions to recent times. This statement from one of the nation's HIV/AIDS policy documents attests to this claim.

> The present multisectoral approach still lacks a legal and institutional framework through which to operate and the sectoral roles of the various implementers are yet to be well defined. This has led to poor coordination, multiplicity of effort and an inability to fully maximize investments in the actualization of . . . objectives.[33]

Other challenges include the weak linkages between various sectors of the economy particularly in development initiatives like poverty reduction programs, and social and legal protection services in HIV/AIDS prevention and treatment programs. While NACA could be said to be a sign of the nation's political commitment to the HIV/AIDS response, lower-level parastatals like the State Agency for the Control of AIDS (SACA) and the Local Agency for the Control of AIDS (LACA), respectively, were established as part of the federal government's directives to expand its HIV/AIDS response and governance to the grassroots. At these lower levels, however, political will and commitment remain severely lacking. SACA and LACA are grossly underfunded and, consequently, suboptimal. In support of this claim, the NSF 2010–2015 reports:

> There are critical shortfalls in technical and managerial capacities in most SACAs and all LACAs. Poor funding of SACAs remains a pernicious and recurring issue. Political interference in coordination structures distorts relationships and linkages of institutions at several levels.[34]

These are fundamental loopholes that undermine the HIV/AIDS intervention chain especially at the lower tiers, for example, LACA, which was designed to act as a direct representation of the grassroots population and established to implement interventions at the community level, a level where the drivers of the HIV/AIDS epidemic are deeply rooted. Another policy text indicated that "there is little evidence of true commitment in many states and local governments as shown by initiatives undertaken proactively to control the epidemic in the various states."[35] In this sense, an underperformance of these lower tiers calls to question the inclusion and representation of local voices, especially the voices of seropositive women in the nation's overall multisectoral response, and if the established mechanisms designed to enable such engagement are deficient. This is an assertation that was corroborated by the representatives of the local HIV/AIDS support group domiciled at the health facility where the cohort of HIV-seropositive women interviewed for this research sought treatment, care, and support. The HIV-seropositive women from the support group decried their lack of access to government agencies and actors, as well as their poor involvement in the planning and design of interventions. Even though a bottom-up model has been deployed in Nigerian HIV/AIDS interventions as most policy documents indicate, these unaddressed issues render this model ineffectual. In other words, effective HIV/AIDS intervention models should go beyond the adoption of approaches that appear inclusive and representative if the mechanisms to render them effective are lacking.

Since 1999 when a more coordinated response emerged, Nigeria has moved through four broad phases of interventions as reflected in its tripartite policy documents: the HIV/AIDS Strategic Framework and Implementation Plan, the National Response Assessment, and Monitoring and Evaluation Plan. The structure of these documents—each with a five-year action plan—shows that Nigeria has undergone three active and almost distinct but connected phases of interventions between 1999/2000–2004, 2005–2009, and 2010–2015/2016 at the time of this research. This timeline is exclusive of the country's initial efforts during the military regime, not considered as an active intervention phase because efforts were erratic and nonstrategic at the time. For clarity, however, I designate and refer to the overall intervention timeline as the early phase, first active phase, second active phase, and third active phase, respectively, as depicted in Table 2.1.

At the time of writing this book, a transition to a fourth active phase of intervention has occurred based on the National HIV and AIDS Strategic Framework (NSF) document for 2017–2021, released in the first quarter of 2017, with a goal to end AIDS in Nigeria by 2030.[36] This document and phase succeeds the NSF plan for 2010–2015 which was extended to December 2016, to allow for the development of the current plan. At this juncture, it is also important to mention that this current intervention phase is not included in the original policy analysis conducted and presented in this chapter.

With increasing knowledge of the epidemic and the need to strengthen the country's response, other supplementary policy plans, for example, gender, have been subsequently launched and established, and sometimes overlapping with a particular phase of intervention. As I mentioned in the introductory chapter of this book, I was opportune to attend one of such policy dissemination meetings on gender, in December 2014 during my fieldwork, where the document on the National Plan of Action Addressing Gender-Based Violence

(GBV) and HIV/AIDS Intersections for 2015–2017 as well as other gender instruments were launched.

Table 2.1. Summary Timeline of HIV/AIDS Interventions from 1985 to 2021.

Early phase of HIV/AIDS discovery in Nigeria, 1985–1998

The era of disbelief, denial, and rejection of Western scientific evidence of AIDS in sub-Saharan Africa, and an initial weak policy response to the disease during the military era which was also a time of political instability. This response was mostly preventative to curb the transmission and spread of the virus.

Phase 1: 1999–2004. 1999 ushered in Nigeria's democratic regime after many years of military dictatorship

This began an active phase of HIV/AIDS intervention with the establishment of the PCA and a national AIDS coordinating body, the National Action Committee on AIDS, with their subsidiaries at the state and local levels. The establishment of the National Action Committee on AIDS was characterized by the recognition of a multisectoral response, given the intersectional nature of the epidemic as cross-cutting different issues that were handled by different sectors. At this time, there was still no access to ARV drugs, so interventions remained mostly preventative with a focus on individual behavioral change.

Phase 2: 2005–2009. Active HIV/AIDS response continued and culminated in the adoption of a strategic plan launched by the international AIDS community known as the "Three Ones"

The Three Ones strategic plan comprised the HIV/AIDS National Strategic Framework Policy (NSFP) plan, one MES, and a single coordinating body, NACA. The National Action Committee on AIDS was transformed into a full agency in 2007, through legislation to further strengthen its coordinating role and overall national response. Interventions were beginning to be a mix of treatment and prevention as ARV drugs were becoming available toward the end of this phase. Yet ARVs were not easily accessible due to physical and economic factors. Gender as an issue of concern was officially launched at this time, in policy documents, through the concept of gender mainstreaming. Gender was, however, mostly defined in categorical terms such that the relational dynamics that exist between men and women were excluded.

Phase 3: 2010–2015/2016.

This phase was characterized by an increasing availability of ARV drugs and a beginning emphasis on the biosocial model of health, alongside existing biomedical interventions. The goal at this phase was universal access to treatment. With increasing availability of drugs came the issue of nonadherence and a focus on the social issues that constrained access and adherence like care and support for the people living with HIV/AIDS. Gender issues continued to be a focus but with marked variations in terms of its conceptualization. Although gender was now constructed in more relational terms, this was not consistent across policy documents. This phase was later extended to December 2016 to allow for the development of the current intervention phase.

Phase 4: 2017–2021.

Current phase of intervention is based on the NSF document 2017–2021, with a goal to end HIV/AIDS by 2030.

PARADIGMS OF INTERVENTIONS

Based on a critical analysis of policy documents, dominant paradigms of interventions have been both biosocial and biomedical. Human rights, social justice, and equity are hegemonic discourses that resonated across policy texts in the first active phase of intervention, and which essentialized a biosocial paradigm. Within this paradigm, rights as a policy discourse was framed as a human entitlement but in practice, it was invoked and targeted as a public health measure to curtail the epidemic in the absence of a cure at the time, rather than its deliberate and conscious adoption on the basis of its constitutional values. As a human discourse, the rights' approach was operationalized against stigma and other discriminatory attitudes that prevented voluntary confidential counseling, testing, and diagnosis by individuals but with an underlying aim to remedy HIV/AIDS under-reporting and other barriers to preventive efforts.

Significant to the biosocial model was that the language of rights was not deployed to challenge the existing structures that violated the rights of marginalized populations and predisposed them to the risks of the virus and disease. Policy documents although invoked rights discourses, they were mostly in connection to preventative approaches that foregrounded behavioral change but left the structural roots of the epidemic unperturbed. In its discursive meanings, the invocation of rights and social justice, although seemed to conjure rights as a legal instrument to protect and preserve the welfare of people living with HIV/AIDS, this model was shrouded by the bias of public health agencies to direct gains toward preventative efforts. The biosocial paradigm and its rights-based social justice approach thus appeared to have been adopted as a contingency model aimed at promoting population health through prevention but by targeting individuals for change.

Although the consideration of rights became more people-centered in the second active phase of intervention, outcomes did not appear to have translated into much substantive improvement in the protection of infected individuals. The weakness in the power of rights to protect the people living with HIV/AIDS in Nigeria could be attributed to the fact that the nation's HIV/AIDS policies did not have the power of laws. As of December 2014, the time of this research, there were no explicit laws on HIV/AIDS, and the related laws, for example, on stigma were referenced within the basic human right laws that prohibit discrimination of any kind.

> The problem is that, at the moment, there are no HIV/AIDS specific laws on the statutes. As legal reforms have been notoriously slow in coming and without the backing of the law, government policy documents can only be inspirational in wishing for an effective national HIV/AIDS response that respects the rights of PLHIV [People Living with HIV] and people affected by AIDS (PABA). . . .

The absence of explicit laws leaves PLHIV extremely vulnerable to the violation of their rights.[37]

The country's weak legal HIV/AIDS framework, however, led to agitations, which prompted the HIV/AIDS Anti-discrimination Act of 2014 that "makes it illegal to discriminate against people based on their HIV status . . . and also prohibits any employer, individual or organization from requiring a person to take an HIV test as a precondition for employment or access to services," to be passed into law on February 3, 2015.[38] Succeeding this law was the sexual offenses bill that was passed on June 3, 2017, with HIV/AIDS-related provisions, for example, the criminalization of HIV/AIDS nondisclosure, exposure, and transmission but one that has been critiqued for its overly broad and vague statutes.[39] While these were steps in the right direction, I have made a detailed argument in chapter 10 of this book that the deployment or application of rights in patriarchal contexts is not in itself absolute in the protection of vulnerable and marginalized women if the negative cultural, social, and religious imbrications of rights are left hidden and intact.

At the beginning of the second active phase of intervention, there was little mention of access to ARV drugs in policy documents, so it appears that treatment was still generally elusive at this time or only available to a few. Access to ARVs as a challenge was underscored in policy documents but defined based on physical, economic, and geographical factors and less on the social processes that produced inequities in treatment. Illustrative of this, equity was mostly conceptualized in economic (affordability) and geographical terms as physical and economic access were the most visible constraints to treatment at the time. Social inequalities in treatment were not central or mainstream and neither was gender. Quality, availability, and delivery of ARV drugs to the infected population appeared to be more important considerations. When women were mentioned, it was as vectors of infection with a focus to reduce the burden of transmission through pregnancy and commercial sex work.

In line with the Millennium Development Goals (MDGs), Nigeria's commitment to universal access to health care underpinned the efforts to improve access to HIV treatment in the third active phase of intervention paving the way for biomedical approaches. With increasing availability and access to ARVs, the need for social support services as germane to improving access and adherence, especially among marginalized groups became visible. This recognition produced a transition into policies and programs that emphasized care and support for treatment in this intervention phase, thereby, reinforcing the biosocial approach to treatment. In spite of the conscious mainstreaming of social dimensions into HIV/AIDS policies, treatment still lacked a clear gender perspective. In addition, social policies and action plans on treatment were weakly framed.

TREATMENT, CARE, AND SUPPORT

Although the year 2010 was targeted for universal access to treatment, gaps in physical access still existed at the time, despite increasing access to ARVs. Other forms of inequalities emerged around access like gender and the lack of care and support services for the people living with HIV/AIDS. HIV/AIDS support networks and other social support systems became important structures leveraged on to improve treatment access and adherence.

Conceptualizations of care were mostly as acts rendered by professional caregivers—healthcare workers, community, and family members of the people living with HIV/AIDS. Providing support to reduce the burden of care for these defined categories of caregivers, thus became a central policy discourse as teased out from related policy documents. Ironically, this is a reversed reality among HIV-seropositive women interviewed, who reportedly are just as burdened with caregiving responsibilities to their families, although in need of care themselves—a lived experience that was absent in policy documents that focused on the thematic areas of treatment, care, and support.

The lack of an explicit focus on HIV-seropositive women as caregivers in HIV/AIDS policies, therefore, necessitates policy actions that recognize the enormous care burden placed on this population especially at the household level and as this constrains women in caring for their own bodies.

GENDER

Policy documents in the first active phase of intervention did not reveal an explicit gender consideration.[40] Initial interventions on gender were weak because of the absolute focus on detection, control, and prevention. At best, the deployment of gender in policy discourses signified a focus on women because the feminized nature of the epidemic gave way to the constructions of female bodies as risky subjects. Such constructions, although implicit, fostered critical national attention to maternal health and other reproductive issues as women's bodies especially those pregnant were perceived as obvious transmission routes. In these instances, gender became synonymous with women, and women were conceptualized as biosecurity agents in the context of the epidemic. The following policy statements are evidence to these claims.

> An increasing number of children are being infected with the virus, through mother to child transmissions . . . by all indications, the HIV/AIDS epidemic has continued to grow largely . . . through mother to child transmission.[41]

> Nigeria shall place the highest possible priority on ensuring nationwide access to antiretroviral medication for all pregnant women with HIV and treatment provided at delivery to prevent vertical transmission.[42]

An active gender plan began in 2005, during the second active phase of intervention, and gender mainstreaming as a formal concept and strategy was officially launched through the five-year NSFP document for the period 2005–2009—a confirmation that gender mainstreaming is a relatively new concept in the Nigerian HIV/AIDS policy landscape. It also partly explains the multiple challenges the country has been navigating around gender mainstreaming as policy stakeholders' responses also indicate from the interviews.

In this phase, the concept of gender had gained more prominence but like the preceding phase, gender was constructed mostly in categorical terms with primary reference to pregnant women, in the prevention of vertical transmissions—mother to child. The application of gender concepts remained vague and obscure, for example, usage of the phrase "gender-sensitive" programs was devoid of details, with little specificity to meaning and strategies. The idea of male involvement in interventions was also referenced but only in the context of prevention of mother-to-child transmissions (PMTCT), and with lack of practical details for implementation.

Gender discourses appeared to shift significantly between 2010 and 2015, with the concept of gender mainstreaming more centralized, and its articulations succinct. Women began to receive focus in HIV/AIDS policies for their self-worth and value as women and not primarily for their social and biological roles in securing the health of the general population.

> In most African societies, women are the homemakers and they play a central role in stabilizing families and maintaining its health. There is evident need to keep women healthy and safe for the sake of their health and the stability of the family.[43]

In spite of these significant improvements, recent policy documents on gender still revealed some antitheses as gender was defined in relational terms but proposed strategies were deployed in gender-specific terms, to include only women and girls. Sometimes, the relationality and intersectionality of gender were underscored, and at other times, they were obscured or elided—a pattern of inconsistency I observed varied across policy documents from various HIV/AIDS-related subsectors and programs. In other words, gender appropriations whether as categorical, relational, and/or intersectional were not uniform across subsectors and programs. A possible explanation for this disconnect is that there are marked variations in the level of gender awareness and knowledge among relevant sectors and subsectors, and this was similarly visible in policy stakeholders' responses. Policy institutions and related HIV/AIDS sectors and subsectors may also not be as collaborative particularly in the aspect of formulating a cohesive gender plan. The lack of a unified and cohesive gender response plan can cause programmatic confusion among implementation partners or policy practitioners who deploy policy guidelines at the level of execution. These inconsistencies mirror the state of a disorganized gender landscape in Nigeria's HIV/AIDS interventions. Also noteworthy was the silence or exclusion of private sector activities, for example, NGOs as they promote or impede the national HIV/AIDS and gender agenda. Existing HIV/AIDS policies and action plans that were available and analyzed lacked a clear reference to the NGO sector and their activities, which have been a strong component of the Nigerian HIV/AIDS intervention landscape.

In general, while the discourse on gender appears to have improved through time with the emergence of a fine policy gender blueprint on HIV/AIDS, it is still replete with flaws, with ambiguities in gender conceptualization, conflicting approaches to mainstreaming gender, and the lack of explicit strategies, as major gaps. Policy plans appear to acknowledge the issues of gender more than having a practical and effective gender plan that proffers solutions.

With a current adult HIV/AIDS prevalence rate of 1.9 percent,[44] a vast reduction from the peak of the epidemic at 5.8 percent in 2001, Nigeria can be said to have shown remarkable progress in its mitigation efforts but critics maintain that the cost of interventions far outweigh the achievements documented so far.[45] The country's multisectoral response to the epidemic remains challenged at all tiers.

In spite of these gains and losses, Nigeria is still on its way to halt the HIV/AIDS epidemic. Beyond the epidemiological drivers of the epidemic, the inaction and delayed response to the epidemic at its onset, a weak political will, inadequate healthcare system, gender and other forms of social inequalities, and the less-than-effective modes of gender mainstreaming into policy plans and actions remain the most visible factors that explain why HIV/AIDS remains a major epidemic in the country.

NOTES

1. Abdulsalami Nasidi and Tekena O. Harry, "The Epidemiology of HIV/AIDS in Nigeria," in *AIDS in Nigeria: A Nation on the Threshold*, eds. O. Adeyi, P. J. Kanki, Oluwole Odutolu, and John. A. Idoko (Cambridge, MA: Harvard Center for Population and Development Studies, 2006), 18.
2. Nasidi and Harry, "The Epidemiology of HIV/AIDS in Nigeria," 18.
3. Jonathan Mayer, "The Geographical Understandings of HIV/AIDS in Sub-Saharan Africa," *Norwegian Journal of Geography* 59 (2005): 7, https://doi.org/10.1080/00291950510020493.

4. Lucy Jarosz, "Constructing the Dark Continent: Metaphor as Geographic Representation of Africa," *Geografiska Annaler. Series B, Human Geography* 74, no. 2 (1992): 112.

5. Susan Craddock, "Beyond Epidemiology: Locating AIDS in Africa," in *HIV and AIDS in Africa: Beyond Epidemiology*, eds. Ezekiel Kalipeni, Susan Craddock, Joseph R. Oppong, and Jayati Ghosh (Oxford: Blackwell, 2004), 3.

6. Ibid., 3–4.

7. Nasidi and Harry, "The Epidemiology of HIV/AIDS in Nigeria," 20–21, 34.

8. Peter Lurie, Percy Hintzen, and Robert A. Lowe, "Socioeconomic Obstacles to HIV Prevention and Treatment in Developing Countries: The Roles of the International Monetary Fund and the World Bank," in *HIV and AIDS in Africa: Beyond Epidemiology*, eds. Ezekiel Kalipeni, Susan Craddock, Joseph R. Oppong, and Jayati Ghosh (Oxford: Blackwell, 2004), 205.

9. Also see Joe L. P. Lugalla, "The Impact of Structural Adjustment Policies on Women's and Children's Health in Tanzania," *Review of African Political Economy* 22, no. 63 (March 1995): 47.

10. Mark Hunter, *Love in the Time of AIDS: Inequality, Gender and Rights in South Africa* (Bloomington: Indiana University Press, 2010), 114–115.

11. Nkolika Ijeoma Aniekwu, "Gender and Human Rights Dimensions of HIV/AIDS in Nigeria," *African Journal of Reproductive Health* 6, no. 3 (2002): 32–33; Lugalla, "The Impact of Structural Adjustment Policies," 47.

12. "Country Factsheets: Nigeria, 2017," Data, UNAIDS, accessed July 16, 2018, http://www.unaids.org/en/regionscountries/countries/nigeria.

13. United Nations, *Nigeria - United Nations Sustainable Development Partnership Framework (UNSDPF) 2018 to 2022* (Abuja: United Nations, 2017), 17, http://www.ng.undp.org/content/nigeria/en/home/library/knowledgeproducts/un-sustainable-development-partnership-framework-2018-2022.html.

14. See Brooke Grundfest Schoepf, "AIDS, History, and Struggles over Meaning," in *HIV and AIDS in Africa: Beyond Epidemiology*, eds. Ezekiel Kalipeni, Susan Craddock, Joseph R. Oppong, and Jayati Ghosh (Oxford: Blackwell, 2004), 181; Anne V. Akeroyd, "Coercion, Constraints, and 'Cultural Entrapments': A Further Look at Gendered and Occupational Factors Pertinent to the Transmission of HIV in Africa," in *HIV and AIDS in Africa: Beyond Epidemiology*, eds. Ezekiel Kalipeni, Susan Craddock, Joseph R. Oppong, and Jayati Ghosh (Oxford: Blackwell, 2004), 90.

15. Penny Griffin, "The World Bank, HIV/AIDS and Sex in Sub-Saharan Africa: A Gendered Analysis," *Globalizations* 8, no. 2 (April 2011): 239.

16. Krishnan et al., "Poverty, Gender Inequities, and Women's Risk of Human Immunodeficiency Virus/AIDS," *Annals of the New York Academy of Sciences* 1136 (2008): 101–102, https://doi.org/10.1196/annals.1425.013; Nasidi and Harry, "The Epidemiology of HIV/AIDS in Nigeria," 30–31; Phaladze Nthabiseng and Sheila Tlou, "Gender and HIV/AIDS in Botswana: A Focus on Inequalities and Discrimination," *Gender and Development* 14, no. 1 (2006): 26, https://doi.org/10.1080/13552070500518095.

17. Durrenda Nash Ojanuga and Cathy Gilbert, "Women's Access to Health Care in Developing Countries," *Social Science and Medicine* 35, no. 4 (1992): 616.

18. Anne Buve, Kizito Bishikwabo-Nzarhaza, and Gladys Mutangadura, "The Spread and Effect of HIV-1 Infection in Sub-Saharan Africa," *The Lancet* 359 (June 2002): 2014.

19. Oluwafunmilayo Josephine Para-Mallam, "Faith, Gender and Development Agendas in Nigeria: Conflicts, Challenges, and Opportunities," *Gender and Development* 14, no. 3 (2007): 411, https://doi.org/10.1080/13552070600980898.

20. Ibid., 414–415.

21. Ibid., 414.

22. Carol Vlassoff and Claudia Garcia Moreno, "Placing Gender at the Center of Health Programming: Challenges and Limitations," *Social Science and Medicine* 54 (2002): 1717.

23. Nalia Kabeer, *Reversed Realities: Gender, Hierarchies in Development Thought* (London: Verso, 1994), 280–281.

24. Ibid., 35–37.

25. Ojanuga and Gilbert, "Women's Access to Health Care in Developing Countries," 615–616; Para-Mallam, "Faith, Gender and Development Agendas in Nigeria," 411, 414.

26. Ojanuga and Gilbert, "Women's Access to Health Care in Developing Countries," 615; Greig et al., "Gender and AIDS: Time to Act," *AIDS* 22, suppl. 2 (August 2008): 2, https://doi.org/10.1097/01.aids.0000327435.28538.18; Nthabiseng and Tlou, "Gender and HIV/AIDS in Botswana," 24.

27. Two categories of documents were analyzed: gender-related policy documents and multisectoral HIV/AIDS policy plans and implementation framework. The documents were analyzed for the ways gender was defined and conceptualized—the ways the language of gender was used and if it somewhat reperpetuates inequalities. The documents were also analyzed for discourses on treatment, care, and support as well as the general framings of interventions and their evolution over time. I make a disclaimer that the policy documents analyzed represent all the available policy documents on HIV/AIDS since the inception of intervention efforts. Rather, the analysis was based on documents that were available and accessible to me through personal online research and handouts from policy stakeholders, at the time of conducting field studies.

28. Gill Seidel, "The Competing Discourses of HIV/AIDS in Sub-Saharan Africa: Discourses of Rights and Empowerment and Discourses of Control and Exclusion," *Social Science and Medicine* 36, no. 3 (1993): 175.

29. Nasidi and Harry, "The Epidemiology of HIV/AIDS in Nigeria," 18.

30. National Agency for the Control of AIDS, *National Policy on HIV/AIDS* (Abuja: National Agency for the Control of AIDS, 2003), 4.

31. National Agency for the Control of AIDS, *National Policy on HIV/AIDS* (Abuja: National Agency for the Control of AIDS, 2009), 3.

32. "Three Ones Agreed by Donors and Developing Countries," The 3 by 5 Initiative, World Health Organization, accessed January 14, 2019, https://www.who.int/3by5/newsitem9/en/; UNAIDS, *"Three Ones" Key Principles: "Coordination of National Responses to HIV/AIDS," Guiding Principles for National Authorities and Their Partners* (Geneva: UNAIDS, 2004), 1–4, http://data.unaids.org/una-docs/three-ones_keyprinciples_en.pdf.

33. National Agency for the Control of AIDS, *National Policy on HIV/AIDS* (Abuja: National Agency for the Control of AIDS, 2003), 7.

34. National Agency for the Control of AIDS, *National HIV/AIDS Strategic Plan 2010–2015* (Abuja: National Agency for the Control of AIDS, 2009), 22.

35. National Agency for the Control of AIDS, *National Policy on HIV/AIDS*, 7.

36. See National Agency for the Control of AIDS, *National HIV and AIDS Strategic Framework 2017–2021* (Abuja: National Agency for the Control of AIDS, 2017), https://www.childrenandaids.org/sites/default/files/2017-11/NATIONAL-HIV-AND-AIDS-STRATEGIC-FRAMEWORK.pdf.

37. National Agency for the Control of AIDS, *National HIV/AIDS Response Review* (Abuja: National Agency for the Control of AIDS, 2009), 14.

38. "HIV/AIDS Anti-Discrimination Act 2014," Nigeria, Center for Laws of the Federation of Nigeria, accessed September 11, 2018, http://lawnigeria.com/LawsoftheFederation/HIV-and-AIDS-%28Anti-Discrimination%29-Act,-2014.html; "Nigeria Passes Law to Stop Discrimination Related to HIV," Update, UNAIDS, last modified February 11, 2015, http://www.unaids.org/en/resources/presscentre/featurestories/2015/february/20150211_nigeria_law. Also see Joseph Onyekwere, "HIV/AIDS Anti-Discrimination Law and Essence of Implementation," *The Guardian*, last modified April 14, 2015, https://guardian.ng/features/law/hivaids-anti-discrimination-law-and-essence-of-implementation/.

39. Bernard J. Edwin, "Nigeria: Senate Passes Law Criminalizing HIV Non-Disclosure, Exposure and Transmission with Vague and Overly Broad Statute," *HIV Justice Network*, last modified June 4, 2015, http://www.hivjustice.net/news/nigeria-senate-passes-law-criminalising-hiv-non-disclosure-exposure-and-transmission-with-vague-and-overly-broad-statutes-in-the-sexual-offences-bill/.

40. For example, see early policy documents like the United States Agency for International Development, *HIV/AIDS in Nigeria: A USAID Brief* (Abuja: United States Agency for International Development, 2002); National Agency for the Control of AIDS, *HIV/AIDS Emergency Action Plan 2001–2003/2004* (Abuja: National Agency for the Control of AIDS, 2001).

41. National Agency for the Control of AIDS, *National Policy on HIV/AIDS*, 2.

42. Ibid., 14.

43. National Agency for the Control of AIDS, *National Guidelines on HIV/AIDS Care and Support* (Abuja: National Agency for the Control of AIDS, 2014), 15.

44. UNAIDS, *UNAIDS Data 2019* (Geneva: UNAIDS, 2019), 76, https://www.unaids.org/sites/default/files/media_asset/2019-UNAIDS-data_en.pdf.

45. Nasidi and Harry, "The Epidemiology of HIV/AIDS in Nigeria," 28.

Chapter 3

The Political Economy and Socioecological Contingencies of the Niger Delta

A general objective of this book is to understand the discursive dimensions of HIV care, by drawing upon HIV-seropositive women's subjective experiences of ARV access and adherence within patriarchal social systems. The analysis utilizes the evidence to shift the normative coding of HIV subjects as individualized risky subjects but as structural subjects, thereby bringing in a structural perspective to understand individual health risks and behaviors. To this end, the preceding chapter provided a gendered context to the roots of the epidemic, within national and global contexts. In this chapter, I narrow down the gendered, social, and political contingencies of the epidemic to the research site, the Niger Delta region, but simultaneously contextualize women's treatment experiences in Erhoike, an oil-rich community, as correlates of the complex interactions of place processes—traditional cultural systems, market-led environmental decisions, and resource use. This region's unique sociopolitical complexities and environmental change make it a perfect case to illustrate how the relations of state, national, and global capitalist forces act on third world spaces, their regional economies, and socioenvironmental and health systems through the apparatuses of domestic policies and transnational corporations (TNCs).[1]

Geographically, the Niger Delta is an oil-producing region that encompasses the natural delta of the Niger River to its left and the Benue River to its right. By this definition, the core Niger Delta region spatially comprises three states; Delta, Bayelsa, and Rivers, which are also Nigeria's dominant petro states.[2] Nevertheless, the Niger Delta has been redefined in geopolitical and administrative terms, and at present, comprises a broader region of nine states that are domiciled in the southern geopolitical zone of the country (see Figure 3.1).[3]

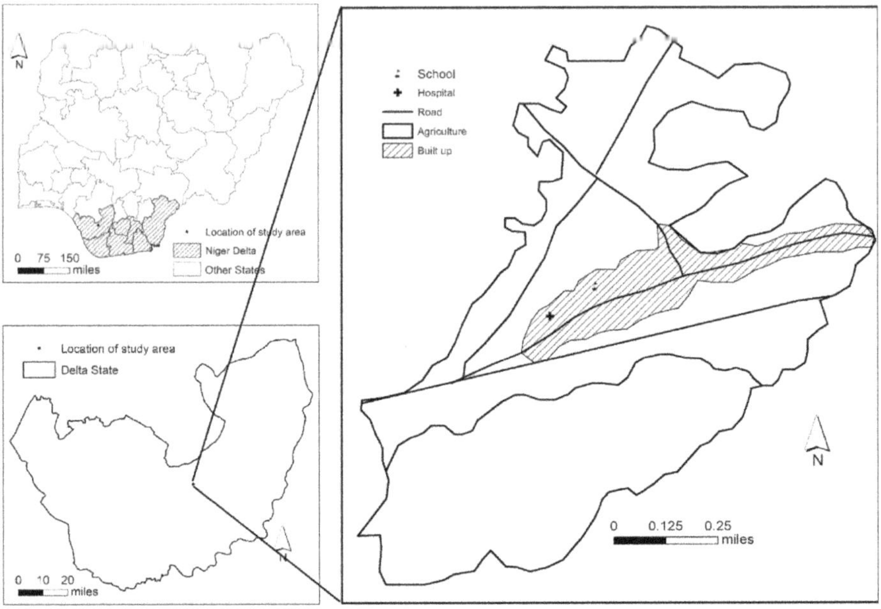

Figure 3.1 Nigeria, states of the Niger Delta region and Erhoike.
Source: Author.

Since the 1956 discovery of oil in the Niger Delta, which also set the stage for huge oil exploitations, its oil-rich lands have become the essential identity of this geography, with the proverbial tag as the region that lays the golden egg because, over time, the region's crude oil resources have become the nation's economic mainstay. Less underscored in popular discourse, however, is that this region is an ecological nidus of rich biodiversity and other natural minerals, with vast agricultural lands, forested regions, excellent waterways, and human resources. Still, the vast amount of crude oil that is mined daily from this region makes Nigeria one of the largest oil producers and exporters in the world. As simultaneously as this region makes the most contribution to the nation's foreign reserve and the federal treasury, of which some are deployed for developmental projects across the country, it is also commonly tagged "resource cursed" due to the high poverty level amid plenty.[4] Oil exploitations through joint ventures with states and TNCs in the region, notably Shell Petroleum Development Company (SPDC) and Chevron, have launched Nigeria into the map of contemporary capitalism, weak state environmental protection laws, repressive and corrupt governance, as well as "internal colonialism" that subordinate the southern geopolitical zone to the north, where political power is mostly domiciled.[5]

From historical antecedents, activism for environmental justice, socioeconomic development, and the right for self-determination by the indigenous population have met with strong political resistance especially by the nation's ruling political elites, who continue to govern based on religious, ethnic, and geopolitical interests to the detriment of the region.[6] In 1995, Ken Saro-Wiwa, a renowned environmental and human rights activist was executed by capital punishment at the behest of the military government over the struggle for resource control and the right for self-determination. His execution is a constant reminder of the ways that redistributive politics, environmental degradation and the accumulation of capital by dispossession associated with the oil extraction economy in this region, often become embodied as suffering, violence, and death. Michael Watts also speaks of this space as a site of resistance that is inextricably bound to the intricacies of the presence of oil resources.[7] In what he popularly labeled as the "oil complex," most communities within the region have metamorphosed into sites of constant violence; power struggle; and resistance to state, national, and global capitalist forces that have decimated the region's ecological environment with little reparation.[8]

From past to present, massive degradation of land, water, and atmospheric pollution have not only destroyed the peasant and agrarian economy of the Niger Delta region but also destroyed the traditional livelihoods of a population of primarily farmers and fishermen who depend directly on the ecological environment for their daily subsistence.[9] In what now appears to be a permanent state of stark underdevelopment in the region, the recurrent incidences of oil spills from pipeline bursts, deterioration of the environment, and vandalism of oil installations by angry youths, there is a constant state of oil-related tensions in the region. Conditions of political turmoil, chaotic restiveness, and violence have thus become the hallmarks of oil-producing communities in the region and are becoming permanent inscriptions on the local landscape as indigenes continue the struggle to procure the needed development in their respective communities.

Significant consequences of this struggle are organized militant groups and their factions in the region, followed by a corresponding militarized response by state and national security forces to subdue local militant movements but primarily to secure oil installations in the region as they became targets of conflicts. In 2009, the amnesty program, which had come as a product of national and global peace talks, and initiated by the federal government to address the region's militancy, had produced a semblance of peace but, over time, had been revealed to be fragile as insurgent and militancy activities resumed soon afterward.[10]

The monumental neglect of this region by the federal government due to inequitable practices of wealth allocation and failure to counter the effects of adverse environmental activities has also initiated a range of social processes that have produced harmful behaviors and choices among the local population, choices perceived as pertinent to negotiate the prevailing circumstances.[11] With high levels of extreme poverty, many women and young girls, in particular, have been thrown into the informal sexual economy where sexual relations are negotiated and exchanged for cash and material goods, with the migrant mobile labor population of expatriates and local oil workers who because of access to oil wealth have become the elites in this region.[12] It is not surprising, therefore, that the United Nations Development Program (UNDP) reported that the highest HIV/AIDS prevalence in the region is among women and young people.[13]

Significant variations of the epidemic exist among Nigeria's six geopolitical zones with prevalence rates showing states in the southern region as most affected (see Figure 3.2). For example, in 2012, Rivers State in the Niger Delta region had the highest prevalence rate of 15.2 percent compared to the national prevalence rate of 3.2 percent.[14] In 2019, the Nigerian HIV/AIDS Indicator and Impact Survey (NAIS) showed that two states in the Niger Delta region—Akwa Ibom and Rivers with 5.5 percent and 3.8 percent respectively—are among the three states with the highest HIV/AIDS prevalence rate in Nigeria.

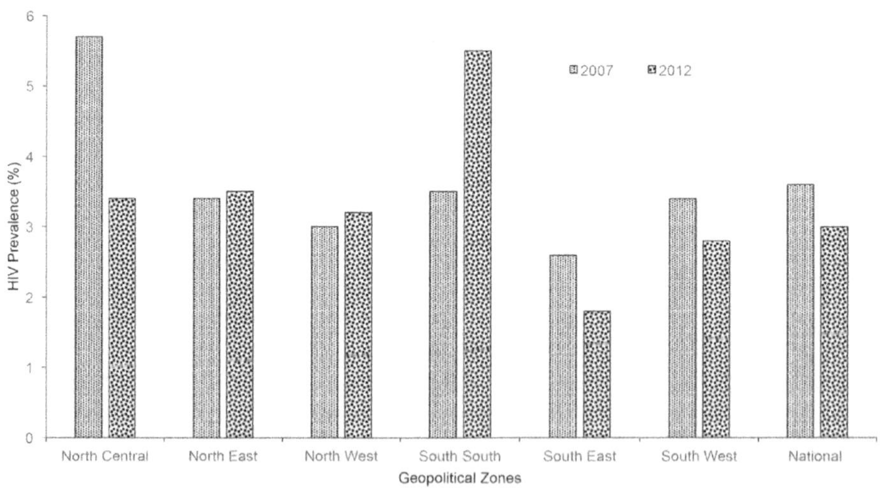

Figure 3.2. HIV prevalence in Nigeria.
Source: National Agency for the Control of AIDS, *Global AIDS Response: Country Progress Report. Nigeria GARPR 2014* (Abuja: National Agency for the Control of AIDS, 2014), 20.

With HIV/AIDS prevalence also linked to extreme poverty, these reported statistics are not unexpected, given the region's unstable socioeconomic and political conditions.[15] In addition to traditional male-dominant structures that position women and girls marginally, a review of existing studies on this region also reveals that women who are traditionally farmers are the most hit with the prevailing environmental conditions as they now have to travel long distances to the interior to find arable lands for cultivation.[16]

In the preceding analysis, I have provided a fairly detailed account of this region's complexities, on the heels of feminist claims that any intellectual attempt to produce a discursive analysis of the embodied impacts of local environmental systems on women, especially in patriarchal orders, must do justice or adequately theorize the ecological and social contexts that impact their lives.[17] To be sure, the varied accounts of HIV-seropositive women interviewed in Erhoike community demonstrate that health experiences and outcomes are inextricably bound to the spatial and social systems in which they are experienced.

Erhoike community, as with other oil-producing communities in the Niger Delta, is a microcosm of the region's oil complex, characterized by a persistent state of insecurity, gun violence, and militarism. As evident in this community and its environs, the physical landscape is dotted with military roadblocks and checkpoints at almost every turn, reminiscent of the volatility of the region. Armed military security personnel (and their paraphernalia) deployed to protect the environment and secure peace have become part of the physical and social landscape. Yet their presence as agents of security is contradictory in many ways. Acts of physical harassment and risky sexual behaviors perpetrated by military personnel who leave their wives and families behind on such assignments have been reported by the locals and were determined as counterproductive to local security as such activities pose threats to human lives and social security. Healthcare landscapes, although by design are supposed to be therapeutic spaces, can thus constitute spaces of risks and vulnerabilities for health subjects like HIV-seropositive women who become bound by these experiences as they access treatment in the community. In the same manner, the health center in Erhoike[18] is also a site of analysis as activities that transpire within it can have as much profound effect on individual experiences of health and well-being.[19]

The notion that individual health risks and vulnerabilities are structurally produced is one that I explore further in subsequent sections. Emphasis is also on the nature of healthcare systems and health service delivery as significant to the healing process and well-being of patients. I explore this theme, which is central to the health geography literature, through the voices of HIV-seropositive women and local healthcare workers at the health center in Erhoike. The geography of health and health care considers as important, not only the locations of healthcare facilities in relation to access but also the actual sites of care, and the modes of service delivery, such that issues that border on experiences of the social dimensions of health care are mainstreamed through consumer self-reports of healthcare provisions.[20] The inclusivity of the voices of health service users, thus, act as significant components of health landscapes because they add new meanings to these sites of care through insights into consumers personal experiences.[21]

The cultural turn in geography, a shift in focus from positivist to interpretive epistemologies in social science explanations, has opened up new frontiers for the socialization of health and healthcare systems rather than a core medical focus.[22] Similarly, the advocacy to essentialize place, particularly its social, fluid, and relational nature, as fundamental to health outcomes has remained a leading theme in the new geography of health, also made possible by the paradigmatic shift to the social aspects of health.[23] As such, a range of geographical research into health and diseases now shows an eclectic use of the concept of place that foregrounds significant shifts from more passive and static constructs—the particularities of place as only physical and empirically captured through multilevel modeling within positivist traditions—to the operationalization of place in metaphorical and nonliteral terms.[24]

These new ways of thinking about space and place have produced the concept of interpretive landscapes, and present place as a complex layering of meanings and histories, and also as an intersection of culture, social, political and economic processes.[25] It is at this juncture that I also invoke the relationality of place and the concept of place as contextual; that is, place as loaded with meanings, in order to situate our understanding of Erhoike community and associated systems like health care, within the sociopolitical and economic productions that have configured it to become a landscape of fear, risk, and insecurity. Within these complex arrangements, it becomes imperative to illuminate how such landscapes reposition women as vulnerable subjects within the realm of HIV care.

ERHOIKE

At first sight, one is greeted by the poor physical condition of this community, the hardly motorable roads (see Figure 3.3) and heavy military presence with multiple checkpoints that house armed military personnel, as one moves further into the town. The feeling of insecurity and fear is also palpable, at least, for a stranger like me on my first visit when I got ordered out of my car by an armed military officer as I made my way into the community. I went through a rigorous interrogation about the purpose of my visit by the military officer and was only allowed to leave when he appeared satisfied with his inquiry. I was further ordered to raise my hands in an act of civilian surrender and trek past the checkpoint to some distance afar, with the driver asked to drive off to pick me at that point on arrival. Whether it was rainy or not, this became my ordeal almost every time I visited Erhoike for fieldwork.

From an insider's perspective, Erhoike is a microcosm of the physical, economic, and traditional cultural systems of most communities in the Niger Delta region. Although I provide details and testimonials that are specific to Erhoike, based on observations and interrogations with the local people and health workers, the accounts presented here are almost a homogenous representation of the subculture of the neighboring communities that are home to many of the HIV-seropositive women investigated.

Erhoike is a small and remote community of about 20,000 persons, who ironically, live in close proximity to a local flow station once owned by the global oil giant, SPDC, the major transnational oil corporation, federally licensed to mine crude oil across most oil-producing communities in the Niger Delta.

As with many oil-producing communities in the Niger Delta, there is a visible deterioration of the ecophysical environment, evidenced by constant air pollution from oil exploitation activities as well as sickly plants and crops that dot Erhoike's physical landscape (see Figure 3.3). The dearth of visible physical development and infrastructure in Erhoike is one out of the many cases of oil-producing communities in the region that exemplify the popular paradox of poverty amid great (resource) wealth. Indigenes are stuck in the recurrent cycle of poverty with high rates of unemployment connected to illiteracy and poor infrastructural development. Although the presence of oil creates a large work force, the community claimed that about "95 percent" of the youths were unemployed and unintegrated into the oil companies. Joblessness, suffering, and living in dangerous environmental conditions have become the bane of many able-bodied youths in this geography.

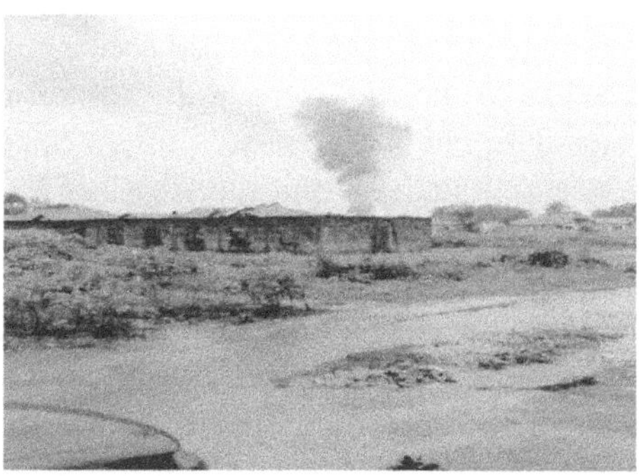

Figure 3.3. Physical landscape of Erhoike.
Source: Author, personal photography.

> Yes, the company neglected us in the sense that we have been crying for long but nobody will put ear to our crying, so what do we do? So we continue suffering. As you can see now, everywhere is dirty yet the oil continues running.—Male, Erhoike community

With a pre-industrial history of mainly agriculture as occupation, the locals have sought alternative livelihoods in artisanship such as masonry and carpentry, and commercial bike riding locally known as *Okada*, in the aftermath of massive environmental degradation from commercial oil activities when their predominantly agrarian culture was no longer tenable. Understandably, local activism and resistant movements against the state and federal forces are based on a protracted history of large-scale structural neglect, and the activities of oil corporations as they have created deleterious environmental effects, which have also resulted in countless civil and social crises pervasive in this community and many others like it in the region.

Reports of internal conflicts and power tussle over local leadership to determine who controls allocations from state and corporate oil entities also emerged among the men during the focus group discussion, and these issues were described to have produced recurrent communal factions and opposition politics, and which I became almost entangled in. In this instance, the focus group discussion was disrupted when the key community informant who had introduced me to the participants left the group due to an emergency. Some other community folks walked in on us and became aggressive toward me and my spouse who accompanied me, with allegations that I was either a spy for the other warring faction in the community or a press reporter representing the government's interest. The latter allegation is also characteristic of the disconnect and distrust between oil communities and government forces or other formally established institutions perceived to be apathetic to the region's cause. It took my spouse *as a man* to mediate the situation, given the marginal value assigned to women's voices, enabling me in turn, to reassure them of my real identity and purpose in the community. Nevertheless, I was warned at the close of the focus group discussion not to return to the community for further data collection as this might spark suspicions from other warring factions and potentially put me at risk if I was perceived to be aligning myself with any particular group in the community. The continued tensions in Erhoike and environs at the time disrupted the fieldwork process such that I was unable to conduct a corresponding focus group discussion with women in the community.

Narrative accounts also place gender relations as highly unequal. Examples of male dominance are revealed through the celebrated birth of a male offspring and in other cases, rejection and abandonment of a female offspring by family patriarchs, for example, at the time of birth in a delivery facility. Interesting, but not surprising, women's positions were mostly mentioned within spousal relations during the male focus group discussion. Reportedly, women are not decision-makers when it comes to the control and distribution of community-based resources. A given example of this is that wealth and other benefits from community-based allocations are generally distributed based on the household as a unit of allocation, with male-heads of households as primary recipients, who redistribute such shared resources to other members of the household, including women. Women's rights are, therefore, limited in both private and public life.

In resource conflict settings like the Niger Delta where distributive and redistributive politics have become the bane of social and economic life, women are further pushed toward the margins of poverty especially at the not-too-visible scale of the household where such politics are further reproduced and enacted. I conduct this analysis with the recognition that a variation exists between men and women in the rights to own, control, and access resources, and this in turn, creates differing sets of life opportunities between the sexes. This gendered pattern in resource control and access on multiple levels is a centripetal force that wields significant influence on all dimensions of women's lives, including health. Within the context of HIV/AIDS where seropositivity is usually shrouded in secrecy, this is particularly important as access to economic and material resources become crucial for the decision to initiate ARTs or for the motivation to seek care.

Undoubtedly, in a community where men are both decision-makers and resource managers, women can mostly exercise their agency in public and private spaces on the authority of men. This notion was constantly reinforced among the male focus group discussants as they strongly invoked their masculinities and rights along religious lines and cultural beliefs that ordain patriarchy as both a divine and natural order of life. Unfortunately, this is a more general perception and reality across the region and country.[26]

Although women in Erhoike are generally excluded from the political realm, they have been used as pawns in resistance and opposition politics, to stage community protests, because of the perceptions of women and girls as docile and less aggressive, and as one of the male discussants stated, the military "does not touch women" as a rule. In contrast, males attract a more violent response from security agents because of the perceived association of violence and aggression with masculinity. Given this perceived military rule of engagement, locally organized women activism are engineered by men, a claim that is corroborated by this conversation with a community health worker.

> *CHW:* Even one [protest] happened recently that all the women were staging [a] fight to the extent that they closed up the flow station for over a week; they were dancing and demonstrating, holding vehicles that are passing to ransom.
>
> *EB:* Just women alone?
>
> *CHW:* Women, they [community] use their women but the men are actually behind it.
>
> *EB:* So it is not that the women on their own have a group that just fights for. . . .
>
> *CHW:* No, no, no. They [community] team up together but they [men] now send their women forward to go and do the revolt because they felt that because if they go together as a team, both men and women, people [members of the military] will take it as a high riot and start shooting but you know with women, people [members of the military] hardly react by shooting; that's why they send their women forward [but] actually, the men are behind them.
>
> *EB:* You don't think that women can actually just go forward on their own and without permission from the men?
>
> *CHW:* No, no, no, no, the men were behind them.

While local women have no authority to autonomously organize and carry out resistance politics, their participation is mandatory when it is called for. Otherwise, they are compelled to pay an imposed penalty fee or fine that is often unaffordable. Female bodies are thus constantly positioned as concrete sites of political power and struggle, along with the diverse social meanings and representations of resource conflicts and environmental change unique to this geography. And by implication, HIV-seropositive women's everyday lived experiences at the personal, household, and community levels are interwoven and constitutive of these complex multiscalar politics.

HIV Care in Erhoike

The health center where the HIV-seropositive women access treatment and care is a relatively small health facility located in Erhoike community. It emerged out of a tripartite agreement with the transnational oil corporation, SPDC, which provided basic infrastructure, administrative services and medical technology; Erhoike community which provided the land; and the Delta State government responsible for health financing such as remuneration for workers. Like most HIV treatment centers in the country, ARV drugs are free in this facility. Cost of access is usually the cost of transportation to

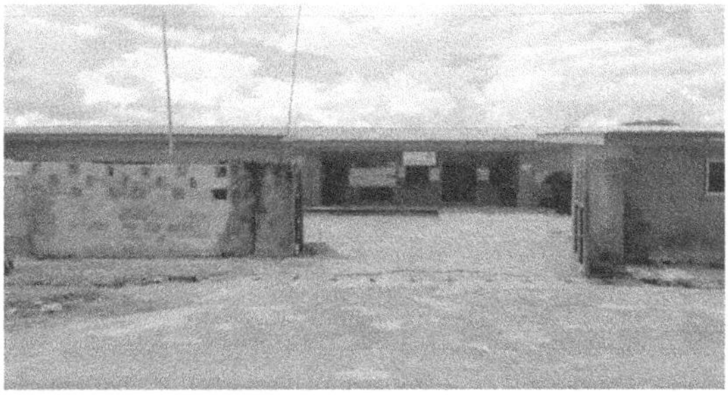

Figure 3.4. Erhoike health center.
Source: Author, personal photography.

treatment centers, and the cost of multivitamins and supplementary drugs for opportunistic infections.

The Erhoike health center was built by the Delta State government as a general purpose medical center in 1995, which in the traditional sense, is a primary healthcare center (PHC). It became a pilot site for comprehensive HIV/AIDS care in 2008, under a project called the Niger Delta AIDS Response (NiDAR), sponsored by SPDC. This project targeted oil-producing communities under SPDC's corporate jurisdiction as part of its social responsibility program.

The NiDAR project was also in response to the country's health system initiative to decentralize comprehensive HIV/AIDS services to the grassroots, for increased access to counseling, testing, treatment, care, and support, especially in high-impact regions like the Niger Delta where travel can be difficult, dangerous, and costly.[27]

Although described as a secondary health facility by its administrator, the Erhoike health center as mentioned hitherto is an upgrade from its original constitution as a PHC. Within the structure of the Nigerian healthcare system, the Erhoike health center may be described as a PHC or a transition between a primary and a secondary healthcare center for the following reasons.

Foremost, PHCs provide the first point of care with referrals to secondary health facilities locally referred to as *General* hospitals. Within the context of HIV/AIDS, PHCs traditionally provide basic services limited to counseling, testing, and diagnosis, whereas, the Erhoike health center provides a comprehensive care package which includes ARV services. To be sure, one of the objectives of the NiDAR project is to counter, in practice, using facilities like the Erhoike health center, the idea that the PHC model is incompatible with the provision of high technology ART programs because such primary care centers are argued to lack certain expertise. Although fraught with many challenges, the NiDAR project appears to have established and sustained a decentralized model of comprehensive ART service delivery at the grassroots through infrastructural upgrade, equipment and commodity supply, as well as capacity-building of local healthcare workers using a health systems strengthening approach.[28]

Furthermore, the Erhoike health center, like other secondary health facilities, is also mostly state-controlled and funded but it also runs self-sufficiently through a drug revolving fund (set up for the center where profit from pharmaceutical sales are reinvested into this funding pool for daily administrative needs); on the other hand, the local government is responsible for the financing and management of PHCs. Similarly, the center receives support from local and international nongovernmental organizations (INGOs) through donor-funded programs. The Erhoike health center's comprehensive HIV service model, funding, and management structure although qualify the center as a secondary health facility, its inability to provide other forms of specialized services characteristic of traditional secondary health facilities and the lack of requisite infrastructure operationally exclude it from this category.

The incessant but irreconcilable communal aggression against the SPDC and vandalization of its oil pipelines ushered in the corporation's divestment program in the communities where they had oil drilling activities and installations, including Erhoike. As part of SPDC's divestment, the Nigerian Petroleum Development Company (NPDC), a public national oil corporation took over the flow station at Erhoike. When SPDC relocated its services, the Erhoike health center then came under the jurisdiction of NPDC. Besides a few administrative changes under NPDC, the structure of the facility and its health services remained unchanged. Under this new dispensation, NPDC performs the administrative functions of SPDC which include obtaining clinical data and general reports from the facility, providing supplemental financial services, and regulating the drug revolving fund. Other functions include facilitating collaborations with NGOs to implement health programs, capacity-building, as well as provision of medical supplies and machinery like blood banks and ambulances, in addition to other technical services.

The rural geography of the Erhoike health center and its remote location at the outskirts of the community have inadvertently proved to be significant influences on the high influx of patients into the facility, especially those seeking to protect their HIV status, due to fear of stigma and discrimination. The Erhoike health center attracts HIV patients of different socioeconomic status, whether local patients from neighboring communities or rich and elite patients from more distant locations and cities, who undertake the long travel to the center for privacy and anonymity. Periodically, these elite patients travel for as long as half a day to a day, to access treatment at the Erhoike facility. In what appears to be a reversed mobility, this pattern of ARV access has created a unique geography of health service access that is opposed to more traditional models of health service diffusion that mirror geographical inequities in health service provision where patients are pulled from the hinterlands into the center or urban areas. Yet what this illustrates is that actual sites of care although physical are loaded with social and cultural meanings, even as such landscapes interact with health subjects in ways that either enable their well-being or increase their vulnerabilities.

Other than its secluded geography, the Erhoike health center also holds a huge attraction for HIV patients because of its nonsegregation policy and practice in HIV/AIDS service delivery. That is, HIV patients receive care like every other patient, with no specially assigned wards and service delivery times for HIV/AIDS services, in order to combat facility-based stigma, which studies show, is a crucial source of HIV stigma.[29] The Erhoike health center has a distinct practice where no single day is designated for HIV/AIDS services, in contrast to the standardized practice in other treatment facilities with designated service days. With this practice, HIV patients receiving care at the Erhoike health center do so anonymously by individual appointments, rather than as a group that converges at the health center on particular days to access services—a practice that may make them easily identifiable. Except on rare occasions when there have been familiar faces among health workers or discriminatory behavior by health workers toward patients, this practice of individual appointments has greatly reduced incidences of health place stigmatization. But as reported by HIV-seropositive women, it is a practice that also has a downside because missed appointments come with verbal queries from health workers and sometimes mistreatment, when patients try to reschedule.

It is also worth mentioning that this practice of ARV access emerged as an organizational policy by the medical director of Erhoike health center at the time, as part of multiple strategies to increase and enhance ART access. Although this policy, as described by the center's administrator, is successful in practice because it engenders HIV-treatment-friendly services and improves access rates, it initially met with resistance by the center's collaborating NGO and partner because it lacks provision within the national

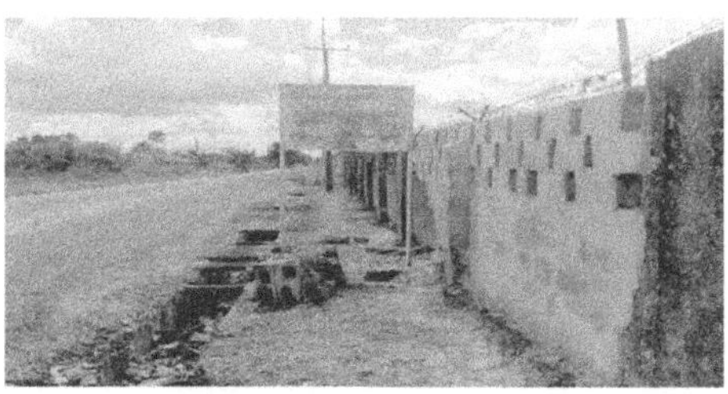

Figure 3.5. Remote location of the Erhoike health center.
Source: Author, personal photography.

HIV treatment guidelines. It is an indicator that too often, standardized and universal guidelines in HIV/AIDS programming are produced at the expense of local needs and the target end-users, and this underscores the need for adaptability and flexibility of so-called HIV/AIDS best practices to fit particular social contexts. Likewise, it also puts forward the claim that healthcare landscapes do not by default constitute spaces of risks and stigma; rather, associated risks are produced. But like the Erhoike health center, there are also possibilities that such spaces can be altered and reorganized to become safer and more therapeutic for health subjects.

Also germane to this geography of ARV access but one that is less foregrounded in HIV treatment discourse is the issue of travel-related restrictions in conflict-prone and volatile regions like the Niger Delta. Sometimes, rumors of war, crime, and conflict undermine sustained access as patients are scared away from visits to the facility, preventing them from keeping up with clinic appointments. Other times, HIV-seropositive women risk their personal security to access care during times of internal communal clashes or face-offs between the military and the communities. HIV-seropositive women living within conflict zones also relocate to safer places, and for some, this increases travel distance and time, which in turn, increases transportation costs as they travel through alternative routes. A common implication is that treatment is discontinued and adherence is undermined, if the increased cost of mobility to the treatment facility is deemed unaffordable.

In one such protracted violent crisis between Erhoike community and government military forces, patients' access to treatment was abruptly halted because restricted mobility produced a temporary cessation of ARTs which caused a relapse for many patients and, consequently, death. Patients who reportedly survived were those who could afford transportation to other treatment facilities, and others who relied on these patients' benevolence to share their drugs. Likewise, community health workers cited personal experiences of physical harassment, molestation, and death threats by armed military agents while they made their way to the facility to assume their duties, due to suspicions that the community health workers were in collusion with the indigenes.

Although these are not very regular occurrences in Erhoike, communal violence and rumors of unrests are fairly common in this region, with treatment access characterized by a lack of consistency while many patients are lost to follow-up. In such physically and socially disruptive healthcare landscapes, alternative strategies for ARV access, especially for vulnerable populations like women are called for. Strategies should transcend simple prescriptions of secondary routes designed to facilitate physical access to health facilities in times of conflicts because these may yet endanger women's lives or prove unaffordable by those already burdened with the usual cost of mobility to treatment facilities.

As the analysis reveals, community health workers constitute an important part of the HIV care landscape. Most of the HIV-seropositive women identified deficiencies in the administration of treatment and also reported dissatisfaction with health workers attitudes which they attributed to lack of awareness and inadequate training of community health workers especially in dealing with infected patients. To illustrate, one of the women narrated an incidence where improperly prescribed medications almost cost her life. Another woman narrated multiple incidences where health workers have wrongly counseled newly diagnosed patients, instilling fear and hopelessness in them. Health workers as agents of care can thus become counteractive to the life-saving ideals and values that they represent.

The politicization of ARV access and reports of unequal treatment of patients by health workers were recurrent in both interviews and focus group discussions among HIV-seropositive women, who claimed that health workers applied a different set of rules to them while patients with higher socioeconomic class were treated better. In making this distinction, the women used the terms "us or we" to refer to themselves and "them" to rich patients. They decried the provision of preferential treatment to patients with material means who are able and willing to make small monetary compensation to health workers to be serviced, regardless of when they show up for treatment, rather than on a first-come-first-serve basis. Some of the women also argued that less-privileged patients experience longer wait times, up to six or seven hours, which usually ends up in conflict with their domestic duties at home as most of them commute from neighboring communities.

HIV-seropositive women also reported cases of patients who did not visit the facility for clinic appointments due to special arrangements with health workers to convey their drugs to them, a behavior perceived to be unfair to patients who are financially challenged or, for other justifiable reasons, are unable to make their clinic days or appointments. For such patients, requests for alternative arrangements to allow friends and families pick up their medications on their behalf are often rejected by health workers who insist that patients must personally come for their medications. While the latter appears to be a standard national ART treatment guideline for facilities in the country, designed to engender provider-patient relationship, such that health workers are able to physically evaluate patients' conditions and their treatment progress when they visit; arguably, it is a guideline that is selectively practiced.

For the most part, this guideline was reportedly violated by health workers among elite patients who never make it physically to the facility; therefore, whatever good reason this guideline was institutionalized, its indiscriminate application negated the original purpose. On the few occasions when such treatment evaluative procedure is reportedly practiced, it is not usually for the benefit of patients but to meet up with the report and documentation demands of the facility's collaborating NGOs. While such inequalities reveal the ways that class differences reproduce and reinforce the inequities that structure women's vulnerabilities in healthcare spaces, they are a pointer to the fact that individual social demographics produce varied experiences of ARV access, with women of lower socioeconomic class likely to suffer more hardships. They also provide insights into an additional category of women who are geographically challenged with ARV access but less underscored in HIV studies; that is, women living in conflict-prone areas.

Based on multiple accounts, other unfair and discriminatory behaviors by health workers include unsolicited and unethical disclosure of patients' HIV status, shouting, yelling, talking down at patients, refusing to attend to patients or administering drugs due to perceived offenses, insensitive comments or statements, and stigma. Health workers discriminatory attitudes not only disrupt the physical process of access, but they also negatively impact patients psychologically and emotionally, as well as the motivation for sustained access to treatment and, by implication, adherence. This has the potential to compromise the recovery process and overall well-being of poor women already burdened with the physical, emotional, and material impacts of their serostatus.

To sum up women's accounts, poor care ethics, lack of professionalization in service delivery, and inadequate knowledge of the pathologies of HIV with its resultant stigma, are reported gaps in HIV/AIDS service delivery. Broadly, these gaps also reveal the lack of psychosocial training for healthcare workers as well as a health system that is weak at its base.

To effectively understand the less-than-optimal levels of ARV access in resource conflict settings is to grasp the complex web of social and environmental risks that patients navigate daily in their quest to seek health care. With women's vulnerabilities also increased due to diminished access to resources, there is a constant negotiation of personal care. The next chapter, as with the rest of this book, demonstrates the materiality of this claim through different scenarios and life experiences of HIV-seropositive women. Individualized constructions of treatment constraints thus preclude systemic factors, rendering them invisible even as they pose the danger of situating women as active sole agents in treatment once drugs have been made available. The path to the health of HIV-seropositive women in risky and violent spaces like the Niger Delta must, therefore, be understood contextually with place-related risks factored into interventions.

Through the geography of HIV care in Erhoike, women's self-reports and experiences also help us to view with critical lens the so-called formal landscapes of health care to unravel the hidden and alternative meanings they hold for end-users and what these symbolize for healing and well-being. Such situated knowledge offers significant utility to researchers and policy makers in repositioning and transforming local health systems.

NOTES

1. People's Health Movement, Medact, and Global Equity Gauge Alliance, *Global Health Watch 2: An Alternative World Health Report* (London: Zed Books, 2008), 14–15.

2. Chukwuma Al Okoli, "The Political Ecology of the Niger Delta Crisis and the Prospects of Lasting Peace in the Post-Amnesty Period," *Global Journal of Human Social and Political Science* 13, no. 3 (2013): 39.

3. United Nations Development Program, *Niger Delta Human Development Report* (Abuja: United Nations Development Program, 2006), 19.

4. People's Health Movement, *Global Health Watch 2*, 171.

5. See Michael Watts, "Resource Curse? Governmentality, Oil and Power in the Niger Delta, Nigeria," *Geopolitics* 9, no. 1 (2004): 58–61, 65, https://doi.org/10.1080/14650040412331307832.

6. Ibid., 51–52, 59–60.

7. Michael Watts, "Antimonies of Community: Some Thoughts on Geography, Resources, and Empire," *Transactions of the Institute of British Geography* 29, no. 2 (2004): 203.

8. Ibid., 209; Michael Watts, "Righteous Oil? Human Rights, the Oil Complex and Corporate Social Responsibility," *Annual Review of Environment and Resources* 30 (July 2005): 9.5–9.8, https://doi.org/10.1146/annurev.energy.30.050504.144456. Also see Watts, "Resource Curse," 62–68.

9. Isidore Udoh, "Oil, Migration, and the Political Economy of HIV/AIDS Prevention in Nigeria's Niger Delta," *International Journal of Health Services* 43, no. 4 (2013): 685–686, https://doi.org/10.2190/HS.43.4.f.

10. Rebecca Golden-Timstar, "Amnesty and New Violence in the Niger Delta," *Forbes*, last modified March 20, 2018, https://www.forbes.com/sites/uhenergy/2018/03/20/amnesty-and-new-violence-in-the-niger-delta/#7188c1d7263f.

11. United Nations Development Program, *Niger Delta Human Development Report*, 4.

12. Ibid.; Udoh, "Oil, Migration," 686.

13. United Nations Development Program, *Niger Delta Human Development Report*, 104.

14. National Agency for the Control of AIDS, *Global AIDS Response: Country Progress Report. Nigeria GARPR 2014* (Abuja: National Agency for the Control of AIDS, 2014), 20.

15. Nike Adebowale, "Nigeria: How Nigeria's 36 States Fare in HIV Prevalence," *Premium Times*, March 19, 2019, https://allafrica.com/stories/201903200030.html.

16. See United Nations Development Program, *Niger Delta Human Development Report*.

17. E. D. Simon, "The Niger Delta Region and the Woman's Predicament: A Study of Kaine Agary's *Yellow-Yellow*," *African Research Review* 4, no. 3b (July 2010), 159–160. Also see Udoh, "Oil, Migration," 686.

18. For example, see Soma Dey, Bernadette P. Resurreccion, and Philippe Doneys, "Gender and Environmental Struggles: Voices from Adivasi Garo Community in Bangladesh," *Gender, Place and Culture* 21, no. 8 (2018), https://doi.org/10.1080/0966369X.2013.832662.

19. Subsequently, and throughout this book, I refer to the local treatment facility where women access ARVs as the Erhoike health center, not the actual name of the facility.

20. Robin Kearns, "The Place of Health in the Health of Place: The Case of Hokianga Special Medical Area," *Social Science and Medicine* 33 (1991): 529–530.

21. Mark W. Rosenberg and Kathleen Wilson, "Remaking Medical Geography," *Territoris* 5 (2005): 23; Isabel Dyck, "Feminism and Health Geography: Twin Tracks or Divergent Agendas?" *Gender, Place and Culture* 10, no. 4 (December 2003): 362–363, https://doi.org/10.1080/0966369032000153331.

22. Rosenberg and Wilson, "Remaking Medical Geography," 23.

23. For example, see Courtney J. Donovan and Ian R. Duncan, "Situating Politics in Health and Medical Geography," in *A Companion to Health and Medical Geography*, eds. Tim Brown, Sara McLafferty, and Graham Moon (Oxford: Wiley-Blackwell, 2010), 176.

24. Robin Kearns and Damian Collins, "Health Geography," in *A Companion to Health and Medical Geography*, eds. Tim Brown, Sara McLafferty, and Graham Moon (Oxford: Wiley-Blackwell, 2010), 16–17.

25. Ibid., 17. Also see Robin Kearns and Graham Moon, "From Medical to Health Geography: Novelty, Place and Theory after a Decade of Change," *Progress in Human Geography* 26, no. 5 (2002), https://doi.org/10.1191/0309132502ph389oa.

26. Wilbert M. Gesler, "Therapeutic Landscapes: Theory and a Case Study of Epidauros, Greece," *Environment and Planning Development: Society and Space* 11 (1993): 171; Kearns and Collins, "Health Geography," 19.

27. For example, see United Nations Development Program, *Niger Delta Human Development Report*, 105.

28. Niger Delta AIDS Response, *Establishing and Sustaining HIV Comprehensive Care Services in Cottage Hospitals in the Niger Delta: Report of the Niger Delta AIDS Response Project* (Abuja: Family Health International, 2009), 1.

29. Ibid., 21.

30. See Herek et al., "Workshop Report: AIDS and Stigma: A Conceptual Framework and Research Agenda," *AIDS and Public Policy Journal* 13, no. 1 (March 1998).

Part 2

EMBODIED ACCOUNTS

Chapter 4

Constructed Gendered Identities: Rethinking and Reconstructing the Notions of Care

We stand together in the shared values of grassroots women caring for their families and communities but against these roles and contributions being detrimental to the health and wellbeing of these women.

—Grassroots Women's International Academy

Between June and July 2007, the Grassroots Women's International Academy and YWCA International Women's Summit was held in Nairobi, Kenya, and was organized around the theme, "uniting communities around caregiving: grassroots women's perspectives on the HIV/AIDS pandemic."[1] An emergent theme from among HIV-seropositive women who were organized from around the continent was the burden of their caregiving roles, which was further compounded by their seropositivity and socioeconomic status. The opening quote in this chapter represents the statement of commitment by the Grassroots Academy and aptly captures the tone and direction to which the central argument in this chapter is inclined.

Progressively, the subject of women and care is garnering scholarly attention in geographical scholarship due to increasing spatial evidence that situates particular experiences of women, for example, health and health care, within care discourses and practices that are sometimes perceived as intrinsic to their ways of being.[2] The intersection of women's health and caregiving, although relatively new and understudied in health geography, provides a significant research frontier to explore gendered patterns in seeking health care and well-being in diverse spatiocultural contexts.[3]

But within the care scholarship, in general, there is not much attention brought to HIV-seropositive women. Even when HIV-seropositive women are considered within the scholarship and in HIV/AIDS policies, they are often positioned as care recipients and not as caregivers.[4] This silencing of HIV-seropositive women obfuscates the problematic tensions and moral dilemmas between caring for their bodies and the bodies of others, the factors that shape the disposition to care for particular bodies, what bodies are cared for, and the conditions in which these take place.

This claim also helps to situate a central argument that I make in this chapter which is that the desire for women to care or develop caring relationships may not always come from a place of nurture. Rather, care is a regulated practice if it is perceived as an obligation that must be performed either to conform to a particular *status quo* or to circumvent certain social and material consequences that may undermine identities and well-being. In this case, I speak of women in patriarchal contexts.

Under conditions of patriarchy where women's autonomies are often stifled in subjection to social, cultural, and gender norms, a commitment to the normative usually takes precedence over other considerations, including their health and personal well-being. Women's minds are conditioned to function in a hierarchical manner that deems compliance with these norms as fundamental to their essence and womanhood. In this sense, protection of the self as a social body takes precedence over protection and care of the biological body. It is within this matrix that HIV-seropositive women must either initiate the decision to seek treatment or otherwise, as access to health services becomes intertwined with other rationalities and not as an action that women can just simply or voluntarily engage.

Ironically, most health interventions construct the body in very biological terms, in stark contrast to women's social emphasis on their body. How we reconcile these seemingly diametric entities through research and policy is of consequence to women's health-seeking behavior. This is also fundamental to non-HIV/AIDS context because oftentimes, policy assumptions about the need for women to make responsible choices in seeking health care too quickly forget the ways that responsibility is structured in patriarchal settings, to make women care for others before themselves.

This chapter is a deliberate effort to engage and amplify the voices and experiences of HIV-seropositive women who are not always given center stage in development thought and practice but more importantly, within care ethical frameworks.[5]

CARE AND RESPONSIBILITY

Fisher and Tronto define care as:

> A species activity that includes everything that we do to maintain, continue and repair our world so that we can live in it as well as possible. That world includes

our bodies, ourselves, and our environment, all of which we seek to interweave in a complex, life-sustaining web.[6]

One obvious advantage of this definition is that it provides a framework that helps to identify a range of processes and practices that can come under the purview of care. The intention is not to minimize the diversity and complexity of care, set limits, or ignore its nuances but to provide a working frame that clarifies the concept under consideration.

A clear interpretation that can be teased out from this definition is the proposition that care is personal yet relational, although, not limited to human relationships. Fisher and Tronto's definition takes a structural yet personal approach to care as maintaining, continuing, or repairing the world that we live in, and where that world could also mean our bodies.[7] In this chapter, I am interested in exploring this dimension of care—self-care—but as it is subordinated to caring for the bodies of others especially within the private domain as constitutive of household and intimate relationships.

Although we can trace the concept of self-care to ancient philosophers like Confucius, and more contemporary thinkers like Michel Foucault,[8] it is still a concept that I argue is yet to receive adequate attention in contemporary care discourses and practices.[9] I also do not engage the concept of self-care in its convoluted and deeply nuanced forms as theorized by Michel Foucault. In lieu, I engage self-care in its most basic form which involves practices that promote the health and well-being of the self.

Fisher and Tronto's definition also conceives caring as both a process and an activity. Care as an activity that is performed, although situates the practice in more concrete and doable terms, must also be considerate of not only the outcomes but also the means to this end. In other words, the process and practice of care should not be viewed as distinct from the resources to perform it but as constitutive and mutually reinforcing, especially in contexts where these resources are women's bodies themselves.

Other essential dimensions of care that I explore are the gendered constitution of care and the notion of care as largely socially and culturally dependent, which have also formed the crux of ongoing theoretical debates and an important focus of contemporary moral development scholarship; that is, the debates on whether care is neutral or subjective and whether care as a practice is based on gender. And in this sense, whether caring is generic to women due to nature, nurture or simply from cultural and societal values or expectations.

In explicating the notion of responsibility, Tronto disagrees with the conventional ideology of likening responsibility to obligation. She portrays these two terms as distinct. To her, responsibility is mediated by a set of implicit cultural values rather than formal rules and promises that demand actions based on prescribed duties or contractual agreements and bonds.[10]

In cognizance of diverse racial, gender, and cultural contexts, Tronto thus proposes a more nuanced interpretation of responsibility, advocating for a greater and flexible continuum in which this term should be deployed.[11] Nevertheless, she maintains that although the disposition to be responsible or to act responsibly may be embedded and regulated by implicit informal rules that sometimes necessitate a feeling or commitment to act, it is never to be conflated with obligation.

Tronto further argues that we are better served when we focus on a "flexible notion of responsibility than we are by continuing to use obligation as the basis for understanding what people should do for each other."[12] In this sense, I gather that Tronto tries to undermine the notion of what I refer to here as *mandatory* responsibility particularly in contexts where the essence of responsibility, as she defines it, can be quickly altered. Tronto's notion of responsibility thus suggests choice and free will. In other words, although responsibility may connote a commitment to perform certain needs, it is still a choice. While this stance makes for a great theoretical argument, its antithesis is often the reality for many women in power-laden contexts where demands on gender roles and responsibilities are perceived as mandatory, and a form of promise and agreement when women enter into marital contracts and informal unions. In this context, whatever dichotomy exists between responsibility and obligation collapses amid highly unequal power relations between men and women.

I agree with Tronto to the extent that responsibility is not synonymous with obligation. However, it can *appear* to be. I make clear, what I consider the fragility and fluidity of these concepts in real time because it is very crucial to the ways that HIV-seropositive women acted upon perceived caring responsibilities within household and private relationships. In this sense, I argue that in particular contexts, the idea of obligation cannot always be solely and rigidly seen from its abstract definition as mandated actions premised on formal rules and contractual agreements. The essence of responsibility, although emergent of unspoken informal rules, may command upon vulnerable bodies the same weight of burden that demands them to act in an obligatory manner. Responsibility can thus assume the form of obligation when the disposition to necessitate action is not a matter of individual choice and when the failure to act is likely to produce unpleasant outcomes for the individual.

With responsibility also comes perceived competence or the ability to act; that is, competence is assumed where responsibility is expected. Responsibility also becomes problematic when there are unavailable or inadequate resources for performance. While I speak of care and responsibility from the standpoint of the marginalized, these practices are not exclusive to this group. Care and responsibility can be appropriated by both the privileged and less privileged but can take on different meanings with each group at the intersection of social and economic power. Socioeconomic power can thrust the responsibility to provide care on the less privileged while the privileged become the recipients of care.

Care can connote a moral good when it is done as an act of responsibility to a need that has to be met on the terms of both the recipient and the provider. It takes a reversed effect, however, if it is conceived and practiced in ways that compel the less powerful to assume a mandatory caregiving role to provide care not for the moral good it portends but for eliciting certain benefits from the receiver. In such instances, the morality of caring can be called to question. I make this claim in the context of private relationships. The debates on professional caregiving as they relate to this claim are outside the scope of this book.

In the rest of the chapter, my analysis is built around these fundamental issues but organized around key conceptual questions that emerged from the stories that HIV-seropositive women shared with me as they described the barriers to their sustained access to treatment, namely; why do women in patriarchal contexts care for others first before themselves? How does care for the self and body become subordinated to care for others? What conditions shape women's caring, whether in a theoretical, practical, or institutional context, and the implications for women's health and well-being?

In proffering answers to these questions, I rely primarily on evidence from HIV-seropositive women's experiences which I juxtapose with the relevant scholarship to illuminate areas of convergence as well as areas where women's actual experiences complicate existing theories of care. I also make attempts to unravel the multiple epistemological and philosophical layers that frame the concept of care and the evolving debates within its scholarship but within a scope that is particularly relevant to this analysis.

Furthermore, the analysis also attempts to trace and showcase how dominant conceptualizations of moral codes like care as restrictive to the private domain have not only excluded the role of men from the type of caring responsibilities appropriated to women but also relegitimized the constructions of care as an essentially female enterprise and as the purview of the less powerful and underprivileged.

A GENDERED MORALITY OF CARE?

Women's constructed identities as "carers" or "caring" as a notion are rooted and interpreted within a moral and ethical framework that has been configured by so many philosophical debates on the ethics of morality and its gendered constitution.[13] The notion that morality is gendered is not new. Throughout Western thoughts and philosophies, the view of a gendered morality has always been subscribed to, along with the notion that women have different moral or ethical capabilities from men, and sometimes less.[14]

Likewise, definitions of what is good, moral, or ethical that are constitutive of values premised on caring—compassion, responsibility, attentiveness, and responsiveness—or which foster meeting the needs of others are traditionally associated with women.[15] But as central and organic as caring may be to morality, theorizations of moral questions have been extremely patriarchal.[16] Questions on moral and ethical codes are thus argued by feminist care ethicists as always cast within a singular universal and patriarchal grand theory that designates moral and ethical codes like justice, fairness, and rationality to men but exclude the notion of caring with its associated affective feminine codes; in addition to simultaneously ignoring the multiple layers and complexities of care through a disengagement of its relational nature.[17]

Moral philosopher Lawrence Kohlberg is arguably one of the greatest influences on contemporary debates on moral development but whose theories met with a lot of theoretical and methodological criticisms. Kohlberg's ideology of morality is argued to be partial and thus objected to because it developed from what is considered to be a biased male sample population.[18] Kohlberg's theory of moral development was critiqued for its elitist approach and hierarchical underpinnings that favored male cognitive abilities, with class and social status viewed as critical to moral reasoning and development.[19] He was also critiqued for the assumption that morality can only be defined in a male's voice. In this sense, Kohlberg was critiqued for conflating the male voice with the voices of justice and fairness as the only moral possibilities, while he implicitly silenced the moral voice of the 'Other' by the exclusion of the female voice, as well as the exclusion of the connections that social relationships make in the moral realm.[20]

Carol Gilligan, another central figure in the scholarship of moral development, in the book, *In a Different Voice* argued that the ethics of morality is also tied to women and connected to their everyday experiences of life. Gilligan's "different moral voice" is therefore definitive of relationships and tied to concrete experiences and activities of care. And while Gilligan may have critiqued Kohlberg's methodology on exclusionary grounds, she falls into that trap, retaining much of Kohlberg's model by developing a theory of the moral voice of the "Other" based on an almost exclusive gender-biased girls-only sample.[21] Along with her suggestion that gender accounts for the only difference in this alternative moral voice, the lack of connections to other countervailing forces such as class, race, and ethnicity, and her implicit feminization of care have also been contested.[22]

Gilligan's view of a gendered morality has been argued to reinforce certain moral boundaries, the public versus private moral divide, which undermines change in the conception of morality and gender roles; for example, it reinforces the notion of politics as an exclusive male moral capability that belongs to the public domain.[23] Gilligan's narrow definition of a gendered care within the private domains of households and relationships, although provides partial explanations to the ethics of care within the realms of power and privilege, does less to view care as possible within the realm of public life—a relegation of care as a secondary form of morality incapable of assuming a centrality around which public and social life can be organized, and by extension political life.[24] Tronto argues that the first task to deconstruct this dilemma is to "recognize that the current boundaries of moral and political life are drawn such that concerns and activities of the relatively powerless are omitted from the central concerns of society."[25] Tronto's three moral boundaries help us to understand how and why the notion of care has been mostly excluded from mainstream moral and ethical philosophies, and by extension, the relegation of care to the private and domestic realms.[26]

The *boundary between public and private life* draws a distinct divide between private and public spheres of life and ascribes the values that define women's morality to the private realm of family and friends but restrictive in the public sphere. The *boundary between morality and politics* is such that mainstream life and political realities largely exclude the values of care because they are deemed to be sentimental or apolitical, with affects and feelings as ethical codes associated with women in the private sphere, as opposed to the public sphere where politics and life are constructed as enacted in rational and desensitized masculine terms. The *moral point of view boundary* considers morality as pure and autonomous, that is, the thinking that morality should be based out of reason and disconnected from affects and feelings, and social circumstances. Viewing morality from a perspective of pure rational reason provides an appearance of the possibility of a universal morality and one that is devoid of context. Thinking about morality this way provides exclusionary grounds for women's morality which is argued to be situated on the emotions and affects of daily life. Desensitized and decontextualized framings of morality provide a lens from which to view the ways that ethical behaviors have long been theorized through a gender-blind lens yet these framings remain gendered because of the ways that traditional moral philosophies define ethical behaviors in patriarchal terms.

These are some of the contradictions that feminists care scholars have challenged and sought to retheorize by injecting women's moral values and practices within mainstream moral philosophies through the ethics of care. Still, when care is theorized, it is abstracted and disconnected from its contexts and practices, largely due to these prevailing dominant philosophical thoughts that morality is universal, distinct, autonomous, and rational.[27] A care ethic theory, however, departs from this autonomous consideration of humans.[28] In contrast, it espouses that humans are "inherently relational" and responsive, and that the human society is centered on this interconnectedness.[29] Care ethics theorists' underscore that care is not only essential to life but also that humanity is organized around caring principles and values.[30] Irrespective of gender, care is constructed to be something all human beings can engage in or are wired to do through relations with others.[31] A fundamental philosophical principle that, thus, underlies care within an ethical care framework is the moral ontology of relationality, which is the claim that the thinking and performance of moral actions are done by the self in relation to others.[32] And the self is conceptualized not as an autonomous, neutral, and objective entity but as a product of multiple identities and subjectivities.[33]

Also related to the ontology of relationality is social relationality, which is highly considered as an intrinsic aspect of care with much value placed on social interdependence particularly as it connects an individual to others.[34] The conception of care and its ability to (re)make the individuals involved in its practice, in morally desirable ways and by extension, the wider networks of public relations that include the social, economic, and political domains have also produced the notion that care should be highly prioritized and valued.[35]

Yet among feminist care theorists, the ethics of care is also very much contested, producing two parallel arguments; caregiving as a rewarding and fulfilling aspect of women's lives versus caregiving as oppressive to women.[36] In practice, the experiences of the HIV-seropositive women investigated straddle this divide.

UNPACKING THE MORAL DILEMMAS OF CARE

In patriarchal settings where women are mostly confined to the private domain, especially the household, their identities and associated roles are usually defined within this space, which traditionally espouses marriage and motherhood. Identities, which are a product of self-internalization, cultural processes and other external human subjectivities within a social system, define the contours of social behavior and ways of being.[37] Extending this logic, identities produce roles and expectations as well as the ways that responsibility is viewed. Where roles and expectations are perceived as organic to ascribed gendered identities in such contexts, they can also be considered obligatory.

Consider the following dialogue with the administrator of the Erhoike health center who works directly with these seropositive women as they access treatment at the health center.

> *EB:* So you talked about nutrition or food as reasons why women do not access treatment all the time.
>
> *HA:* That can be one of the factors because if you look well, you will know that the men are more fed than the women.
>
> *EB:* How?

HA: I will explain to you. A woman that will cook a pot of food, the best fish inside the pot of food, she will serve it to the man to eat, but she is ready to eat *pomo* [cow skin which is the least nutritional part] and all sorts of rubbish, all to satisfy the man, and even when you look at the packed cell volume (PCV) of women in the hospital, you will see men having fifty-something as PCV. You will hardly have a man having forty-something as PCV but women are having thirty-something. Even though we say that the factor of menstruation is there, we still observe that men feed well more than women, so that factor is actually affecting women.

EB: Is it because they are men, and women are women, so men are actually supposed to eat the bigger portion?

HA: [Laughs] I don't really know but that is what is happening. We women, we try to please our men [still laughing] by starving ourselves but in the real sense, we are suffering. Like now, we have also found out that at times, if the woman is infected with HIV, and the man is equally infected with HIV at the same time, the woman will die first, and the man is still alive.

EB: Why?

HA: That is to say that the immune system of the man is higher than that of the woman because the man is eating more, unless on the condition that we find out that the man is a womanizer. If the man is a womanizer, his immune system will drop very fast but if the man is not a womanizer, [and] if he is eating well and holding firm to himself [abstinence or being faithful to his partner], you will see the man healthy for a long time. Nothing [bad] will happen, but for the woman, any little thing, the woman drops [dies].

EB: Are you saying that most times, the woman dies first?

HA: [Yes] first before the man.

EB: So does that mean the man is receiving more care than the woman?

HA: Yes exactly, the man is eating more, eating better, good food and is not facing much stress like the woman.

In Nigeria, women's identities and notions of self are deeply structured by patriarchal conventions and reinforced by cultural laws that legitimize femininity through traditionally defined roles in the domestic and reproductive realms.[38] Even more profound is that this system is socially and politically organized around the core religious principles of Christianity and Islam.[39] Submission to male dominance and the association of the virtues of altruism, nobility, rightness, and self-sacrifice with women are upheld as profound spiritual truths and cultural values.[40] Women have, thus, been conditioned to accept such ethical values as intrinsic aspects of their identities with the essence of womanhood constructed in part, as the ability of a woman to put others before herself.[41]

As we see in the excerpt above, care and responsibility are thus performed within this realm of maternal affects and virtues where the needs of husbands and immediate family members especially children are prioritized and available resources distributed respectively. In situations of inadequate household resources, a triage of care emerges in the household—care for the self, care for partners, and care for children—and choices will have to be made. Most often, women do not choose themselves.

Two cognitive schemas significantly govern the relation of care as a sacrificial behavior at the intimate and household levels; that is, care performed to secure personal security and relationships, and a "silencing" or "suppressing" of the self and personal needs to avoid conflicts.[42] Often the disposition of women (usually the subordinate partner) to care within these relations is marked by their socioeconomic dependencies and vulnerabilities. To establish social and economic securities within the household, the performance of care becomes an imperative to legitimize women's identities as wives or mothers, which also forms the basis for which resources can be claimed within this space.

For a woman, therefore, the household can be a site of security or chaos depending on the decision she makes whether to be subservient to her ascribed identities and roles or otherwise—a decision that is also influenced by the perception of a lack of or limited alternatives outside the household. HIV seropositivity and its concomitant social implications are perceived to further constrict available opportunities, as this statement indicates.

> I have a friend that the husband maltreats. He will even lock the door of their home against her but because of her condition, she is HIV positive and the man is not, she said that anything that the man tells her to do, she will do because the man can ask her to leave [the home or marriage]. And if he does that, according to her, it is not easy to get a man so she will have to remain in the marriage and endure.—[Translated] HIV-seropositive woman

Oftentimes, women may consider adapting to male control or dominance, endure abuse, hardships, or other forms of violence to remain within this traditional unit of the household than to relinquish their identities as wives and, sometimes, their economic security because of the associations of women and their socioeconomic securities as mostly possible within the boundaries of marriage and the household. At the private and intimate levels, although women may play the role of caregivers, care practices are produced within a range of processes that are defined by the terms or nature of relationships but under the influence of prevailing broader forces that produce unequal power and social hierarchies between men and women. Care as a moral imperative ends up being performed under conditions of power imbalances and male domination which can quickly alter the essence of care, making it a site of women's oppression.

Women's caring, therefore, although not inherently bad because it can be a fulfilling experience indeed, as have been argued;[43] I contend, nevertheless, that women's disposition to care can become constant iterations between the realms of voluntary compassion and mandatory responsibility in the present context. Care should not be a venture that is practiced at the whim of the powerful especially in intimate relationships without due considerations to the conditions of service or the welfare of those who provide it.

Limited options can quickly become no options when women are HIV-seropositive but feel obliged to stay as carers in and of deeply damaging relationships with men. Care as an activity by the subordinated and less powerful can thus be enacted as an obligatory response to fulfill the needs of the more powerful and privileged, and a form of patriarchal control and health constriction especially when the caregiver is disadvantaged in terms of resource ownership and control. In other words, the process and terms of care become defined from the standpoint of the powerful who may be the care recipient and not from the caregiver who is performing the activity. Care practice in such contexts can then become a debilitating experience as this HIV-seropositive woman attests to in the following statement which has been translated from Pidgin English.

> Do you know what happened, even our sister here [referring to one of the two leaders of the HIV support group who also works as a home-based caregiver] is aware of this experience because I was sick during this time. . . . I had managed to save money for two months to come collect antiretroviral drugs for my husband. . . . I came to the health facility that day and it even rained on me so that I caught a cold. Still, I waited here [at the facility] from 8 a.m. to around 2 p.m. or 3 p.m. . . . that day. I waited until I was tired and to the extent that my neighbors started calling me that my children were home from school and they needed to eat. And since my children are not used to eating from other people, I had to leave and rush back home without the drugs. The following morning, I got here at 6 a.m. and I started crying because in spite of all the stress the previous day, I was unable to go home with the drugs. . . . If I do not have the mind that I need to do this [go through this stress] to save my husband's life [who is also HIV positive] in order to prolong his life, would I have come back the next day?—HIV-seropositive woman

This is one such illustration that aptly demonstrates the care dilemma that many HIV-seropositive women experience daily at the household level. Although HIV-seropositive herself, she is expected to juggle the responsibility of taking care of the husband and children while relegating her own care, and in this case, to the detriment of her health and well-being. Care for others can thus be a disenabling experience for HIV seropositive women who need care themselves but must first care for others.

Also, this foregrounds the conflict between a care for the self and a care for others that women must daily navigate, especially where seropositivity is at force and treatment at stake. In reality, self-care is always present as a need but may be relegated to the ethical decision to care for others. Ability to perform self-care is, therefore, entangled and regulated by a web of external forces that may either enable or impede it. Most of the HIV-seropositive women recognized and articulated the need for self-care but they seemed oblivious of the tensions between existing negative societal norms and their ability to care for themselves; hence, this connection was not explicit in their personal accounts. Expectedly, there was a lack of resistance to these harmful norms but only the subtle expressions of concern on finding appropriate strategies to manage their health care (with respect to sustaining access to their ARTs) with what was considered their care obligations, especially around spousal and childcare. In other words, besides gender, household relations embody biological and emotional connections like motherhood which come with responsibilities and the (in)voluntary commitment to care.

Care and responsibility, thus, form an important binary in this relational ethical model. The embodied accounts of HIV-seropositive women also compel us to think about the notion of care as a material and concrete expression of responsibility that is entangled in a web of biological, social, religious, economic, and cultural factors that are deeply contextual. Like popular claims by feminist care theorists, this book reechoes the need to not understand and interpret care solely within a collection of universal truths and principles but also within specific spatial contexts.

One of the practical implications of the relational model of care, I argue, is that it not only casts moral actions mostly in the context of "others," but it also reinforces this as very normative. Care in relation to the self is, thus, less foregrounded as a moral imperative. Within this model, caring as a moral virtue is mostly centralized in the context of relationships as performing a moral good is usually conceived in relation to others. Albeit unintentionally, a relational model of care, therefore, establishes the context for which morality is to be enacted as usually within relations to others outside of the self. Self-care is thus less featured as an ethical imperative because it is inadvertently silenced in this moral realm of responsibility and care actions. And in socioreligious contexts where notions of selflessness and altruism associated with women are preeminent, care that is foremost directed at the self may be perceived as self-seeking or transgressing these socioreligious principles. Again, consider the following narrative:

> *HPW:* I will use myself as an example. Even though it was my husband that infected me [with HIV] and he is supposed to feel sorry, he still doesn't feel sorry. He still has the full belief that even if I leave today, someone else [another

woman] will come in, you understand? And my kids, I can't say I am a single parent because I don't just want to accept it but most of the responsibilities fall back to me.

EB: But you people are still married?

HPW: Yes

EB: He doesn't take care of all that?

HPW: He does not. It is only when he maybe, how will I put it? When I get really pissed off and I try to leave the house for some time, that is when he knows he will understand. That is when he knows that he has a responsibility to do. But immediately after that, if I return back to the house, he still does the same thing [neglect her and the kids], so they [the society] will tell you, "na you born the pikin" [this is in Pidgin English but directly translated as "you are the one who gave birth to the children"] so it is your responsibility to take good care of them and make sure they are comfortable. And you know, every woman, there is no woman that will say after having your baby, you can't even provide what [you] want for him or her. You know, you will want to do everything to make your kids comfortable and even without the man's help because you cannot abandon your own children.

EB: Is this something relating to maternal instincts or women as caregivers as opposed to men who feel that the responsibility of taking care of children is actually the women's?

HPW: Yes, yes.

EB: So how does this conflict with your accessing treatment?

HPW: Like my husband, [he] will not even give me money to come pick up his [ARV] drugs, even transport [fare], he won't do it. I am the one that does that and I am the one that ought to pick up his drugs. The only thing he will tell me is, thank you; that is just it.

EB: And not that you have so much [money]?

HPW: No [but] I will have to, it is a must, I will have to do it because I will want him to still stay alive for the kids.

This dialogue captures my initial claims of mandatory responsibility and the ways women feel compelled to perform ascribed responsibilities, while men consider responsibility as a choice. It also depicts the extra burden placed on HIV-seropositive women who by societal default and seropositivity are already vulnerable, yet are conferred with the dual burden to act as both caregivers and providers to their families, while navigating their seropositivity because of harmful patriarchal customs.

In most parts of Nigeria, including the Niger Delta region, where children's biosocial ties are usually constructed in relation to the mother, childcare is deemed as an essential purview of the mother and less the father because of women's biological anatomies and reproductive nature, while men are culturally ascribed the status of providers. In some cases, this breeds irresponsibility on the part of fathers who absolve themselves of any social and even financial responsibility in the upbringing of their children. Such ambivalence in societal standards breeds a crop of men who care less to live up to their provider status. While such masculine behavior is generally condemnable, it is tolerated compared to when women are the perpetrators of such irresponsibility.

Customarily and legally, men reserve most of the rights to their children and can claim paternity at will whether or not they perform their paternal duties because patriarchal customs automatically confer progeny and lineage descent to the male parent, irrespective of situations where the mother has been largely responsible for the children's upbringing. Misguided conceptions of the feminization of care and responsibility in this spatial context have, thus, not only reified essentialized notions of maleness that are unconnected to the schema of care, but they have also (re)produced "male irresponsibility" and other unhealthy forms of masculinity.[44]

RETHINKING CARE

Constructions of care as an ontological female ethic also obscure the power relations and social tensions wherein care and responsibilities are produced and practiced in patriarchal systems. Not surprising, caregiving is very rarely perceived as a burden for women in this context because such essentialized biological and social constructs produce an erroneous assumption of agency. While I favor the arguments for the connectedness of human nature, I make the claim that theoretical and cultural emphases on the relational nature of care may also albeit unintentionally reinscribe the oppressive relations in which care in the context of others takes place, if the conditions and social forces that violate the moral codes of care are not actively resisted and reworked.

As I previously stated, the care ethics scholarship has made significant contributions in destabilizing mainstream gendered notions of care and breaking down the nature-nurture binary that designates caregiving to only women by its fundamental claims that as humans we are all wired to be empathic, relational, and responsive.[45] And that humanity has achieved progressive growth over the years because it has organized moral life around the values of care.[46] Although this normative emphasis by care scholars on valuing care makes an important ethical intervention, I argue that a simple valorization of care as what all individuals do or are predisposed to do can have the reverse effect of not only devaluing women who do all the care work but also the work that they do within patriarchal contexts.

Bringing recognition and value to women's care work by itself is laudable but it may serve to reinforce a traditional moral trap for women—that is, women's commitment to perform care work and not because the conditions for performance have improved. Emphasizing the value of women's care work is much advocated for but it does not diminish the challenging conditions in which such care work is performed and the personal sacrifices and hardships that women often endure.

Frequently, the dominant narrative in the general scholarship on care has been to assign social and material value to care work but what is less foregrounded are the processes and conditions in which care is practiced especially as a personal responsibility in the private domain. Agitations for the recognition of care work and the conditions of performance have been mostly focused on professional caregiving and less on the provision of individualized care in the not-too-visible realms of the household and interpersonal relationships, especially by HIV subjects who may themselves be vulnerable and require care. Women's self-care is, thus, almost overlooked and less centralized in the cultural and theoretical discourses of care, regardless of the well-known fact that women who must care for others must first care for themselves. While a relational care is ethical, its practice must not be at the expense of those who perform it.

To be fair, feminist care ethicists have argued against the relationality of care associated with the subordinate status of women in patriarchal societies as inorganic to the kind of care they advocate for. For example, in a 2011 interview, Carol Gilligan mentioned that a *feminist ethic* of care is a resistance to patriarchal injustices that inscribe care as a matter of obligation for women in interpersonal relationships.[47] Within patriarchy, therefore, care becomes a *feminine ethic* but a *human ethic* within democratic frameworks.[48] Hence, it has been espoused that the ethics of care do not suggest that humans are solely constitutive of the relations they are in or stuck with them if they are unwholesome.[49] Rather, "such persons can and should evaluate and shape these changing relations autonomously, while recognizing that they are part of who we are. This conception of the person is compatible with the priority of care" but not as the isolated and autonomous individual who is dominant in traditional moral philosophies.[50] In other words, there is a recognition of an autonomous self (but not to be conflated with separateness referenced by mainstream moral development theorists) that is relational and has the ability to act independently or *autonomously* to remake care relations in morally desirable ways. To be sure, this autonomous self has been defined by care ethicists as one who is freely capable of pursuing her own projects.[51]

These disclaimers of the oppressive relations of care clearly recognize the influence of patriarchy and other contextual factors as reconfiguring the ontology of care.[52] While such rationalizations pay due considerations to patriarchal contexts, they are somewhat reductionist and problematic because they do not fully reflect the realities of many women whose personhood are intricately dependent on the relations that they are cautioned to extricate from. The extent to which women in patriarchal societies can recognize their oppression within caring relations and disentangle themselves or shape them *autonomously* may vary by how much these women are immersed within their cultures, and also by other indicators like education and socioeconomic power. But because inequalities are not only material but also ideological, the assumption by feminist theorists that *all* women within undesirable relations in oppressive cultures can first, recognize their oppression and appropriately evaluate their situations based on an idealized notion of caring is thus, inherently contradictory. This can only be true if we erroneously assume that caring in such contexts for the most part is an activity or practice that women can voluntarily engage in and disengage from when the situation is unfavorable to them.

In reference to my previous argument on constructed identities, ascribed roles, and responsibilities, women in general tend to define themselves primarily in the context of their relationships with men and children. On this ground, such notions of agentic autonomy ignore this subliminal conception of the self as sacrificial within these connections and relationships. While HIV-seropositive women's experiences reveal an implicit need to pursue self-care and a desire for healthy relationships, their accounts depart from this construction of personhood with an assumed "agentic autonomy to pursue their personal wellbeing" outside these oppressive relations.[53] To illustrate with one of Michel Foucault's basic concepts of care, self-care is a sign of individual freedom because only the subject has the capacity to provide it.[54]The lived experiences of HIV-seropositive women thus illuminate the idea of the particularism and situatedness of care as unique to specific spatial contexts and also challenge critical theorizations of care that appear contextual but pay only partial attention to context.

At this juncture, I make a personal disclaimer that my intention is not in any way to legitimize the negative discourses and harmful practices of care in patriarchal contexts like Nigeria but to illuminate the experiences of women because they exist. This discourse is also an attempt to valorize the experiences of a group of women who have not been centralized in the discourses of care even though they form a crucial part of it with the significant contributions they make daily in bringing care to others. It is intended that the consciousness and legitimacy of these women's experiences will especially help in shaping the way we do health interventions which are critical to women's lives as, ironically, HIV-seropositive women are not provided adequate care in formal healthcare landscapes despite their caregiving roles.

HIV/AIDS policies and interventions are yet to actively consider the caregiving roles of HIV-seropositive women at a personal level and their contributions to the HIV care landscape as well as communities; for example, through home-based care and follow-up services that they render to other infected patients as well as community-based prevention efforts that develop HIV/AIDS-resilient communities. How these care activities may constitute a burden for HIV-seropositive women and further challenge their health and well-being receive little to no attention in policy discourses and interventions. Again, this obvious neglect may be attributable to the taken-for-granted care-giving roles of women due to the conception of care as organic to women. Care as practiced by women under dire conditions can thus be detrimental to sustained treatment access and adherence and, therefore, inimical to treatment initiatives.

While the performance of care in power-loaded contexts can be a truly dehumanizing experience for women in general, it is even more so for women whose seropositivity further complicates their already-marginal status because seropositivity, as we hear in HIV women's own voices, does not in any way preclude them from performing what is supposedly their caring "responsibilities." Rather, biomedical self-care becomes problematized as a burden and when not performed and timely too can have the dire implication of not only costing them their health but also costing them their lives.

The voices of HIV-seropositive women should thus compel us to rethink existing theoretical discourses of care and to search for constructive ways that such discourses can meaningfully be engaged to improve the lives of vulnerable women whose seropositivity is not a safety net against harmful care practices in patriarchal contexts. In this sense, I argue for an understanding of the everyday real implications of such hegemonic discourses even if it is only in terms of the social consequences for the people they affect. This approach necessitates a mindfulness of the need to theorize social issues not only from a critical lens as academic outsiders but also from an indigenous insider's perspective with full attention to the diverse cultural meanings and real conditions in which our theorizations are embedded.[55]

Importantly too, the overemphasis on the concept of care as always relational with less emphasis on self-care may also unintentionally continue to misinform traditional discourses of care in patriarchal settings. Contextual analysis of care must take full consideration to the diversity of its experiences, especially in cultural contexts where male dominance is at force, with the recognition that the same oppressive relations that compel women to care may also constrict their ability to recognize these circumstances or the agency to act autonomously for change. I further this line of argument in the next two chapters, through nondisclosure decisions on seropositivity and local discourses of empowerment, respectively, where HIV-seropositive women although desire to be empowered, demonstrate an unwillingness to challenge the existing social *status quo* in their most intimate relationships either because of perceived normalcy or feared consequences that such disruptions may yield.

NOTES

1. Huairou Commission, *Uniting Communities around Caregiving: Grassroots Women's Perspectives on the HIV/AIDS Pandemic: A Report from the Grassroots Women's International Academy and YWCA International Women's Summit, Nairobi, Kenya* (Brooklyn: Huairou Commission, 2007), 47, https://huairou.org/wp-content/uploads/2016/06/Huairou_YWCA_Report.pdf.

2. See Isabel Dyck, "Feminism and Health Geography: Twin Tracks or Divergent Agendas?" *Gender, Place and Culture* 10, no. 4 (December 2003): 362–363, https://doi.org/10.1080/0966369032000153331; Victoria Lawson, "Geographies of Care and Responsibility," *Annals of the Association of American Geographers* 97, no. 1 (2007): 7; Isabel Dyck and Parin Dossa, "Place, Health and Home: Gender and Migration in the Constitution of Healthy Space," *Health and Place* 13 (2007), https://doi.org/10.1016/j.healthplace.2006.10.004.

3. Dyck, "Feminism and Health Geography," 361–362.

4. For example, see Joan C. Tronto, *Moral Boundaries: A Political Argument for an Ethic of Care* (New York: Routledge, 1993), 144.

5. Huairou Commission, *Uniting Communities around Caregiving*, 6, 11.

6. Berenice Fisher and Joan C. Tronto, "Toward a Feminist Theory of Care," in *Circles of Care: Work and Identity in Women's Lives*, eds. Emily K. Abel and Margaret K. Nelson (New York: State University of New York Press, 1990), 40.

7. Iva Apostolova and Elaina Gauthier-Mamaril, "Care and the Self: A Philosophical Perspective on Constructing Active Masculinities," *Feminist Philosophy Quarterly* 4, no. 1 (2018): 2, https://doi.org/10.5206/fpq/2018.1.2.

8. See Daniel K. Gardner, *The Four Books: The Basic Teachings of the Later Confucian Tradition* (Indianapolis, IN: Hackett Publishing Company Inc., 2007), 4; Michel Foucault, *Subjectivity and Truth Ethics: Subjectivity and Truth* (New York: The New Press, 1997), 89.

9. But see scholarship in social works that imbricates professional caregiving with self-care. For example, Merlinda Weinberg, "The Ideological Dilemma of Subordination of Self Versus Self-Care: Identity Construction of the 'Ethical Social Worker'," *Discourse and Society* 25, no. 1 (2014), https://doi.org/10.1177/0957926513508855; Sara K. Bressi and Elizabeth R. Vaden, "Reconsidering Self Care," *Clinical Social Work Journal* 45, no. 1 (2017), https://doi.org/ 10.1007/s10615–016–0575–4.

10. Tronto, *Moral Boundaries*, 131–133.

11. Ibid.

12. Ibid., 133.
13. Ibid., 61–63.
14. Ibid., 62.
15. Ibid., 3; Peta Bowden, *Caring: Gender-Sensitive Ethics* (New York: Routledge, 1997), 6.
16. Tronto, *Moral Boundaries*, 3–4.
17. See Bowden, *Caring*, 5–11.
18. Carol Gilligan, *In a Different Voice: Psychological Theory and Women's Development* (Cambridge, MA: Harvard University Press, 1982), 18.
19. Tronto, *Moral Boundaries*, 67–76.
20. Gilligan, *In a Different Voice*, 18–22, 28–30.
21. Tronto, *Moral Boundaries*, 81.
22. Ibid., 81–85, 91.
23. Ibid., 86–96.
24. Ibid.
25. Ibid., 20.
26. Ibid., 6–11, for the three moral boundaries as summarized below.
27. See Ibid., 27, 52–56.
28. Virginia Held, *The Ethics of Care: Personal, Political, and Global* (New York: Oxford, 2006), 13.
29. Carol Gilligan, "Carol Gilligan," *Ethics of Care*, last modified June 16, 2011, http://ethicsofcare.org/carol-gilligan/.
30. Held, *The Ethics of Care*, 10; Tronto, *Moral Boundaries*, 62.
31. Gilligan, "Carol Gilligan." Also see Linda Thompson, "Conceptualizing Gender in Marriage: The Case of Marital Care," *Journal of Marriage and Family* 55, no. 3 (August 1993): 559.
32. Lawson, "Geographies of Care and Responsibility," 4. Eva E. Skoe and Rhett Diessner, "Ethic of Care, Justice, Identity, and Gender: An Extension and Replication," *Merrill-Palmer Quarterly* 40, no. 2 (April 1994): 284.
33. María-Cristina Díaz Garcia and Friederike Welter, "Gender Identities and Practices: Interpreting Women's Entrepreneurs' Narratives," *International Small Business Journal* 31, no. 4 (June 2013): 386–387, https://doi.org/10.1177/0266242611422829.
34. Lawson, "Geographies of Care and Responsibility," 3.
35. See Held, *The Ethics of Care*, 133–136.
36. Emily K. Abel and Margaret K. Nelson, "Circles of Care: An Introductory Essay," in *Circles of Care: Work and Identity in Women's Lives*, eds. Emily K. Abel and Margaret K. Nelson (New York: State University of New York Press, 1990), 6.
37. Garcia and Welter, "Gender Identities and Practices," 386–387.
38. Oluwafunmilayo Josephine Para-Mallam, "Faith, Gender and Development Agendas in Nigeria: Conflicts, Challenges, and Opportunities," *Gender and Development* 14, no. 3 (2007): 409, https://doi.org/10.1080/13552070600980898; Nkolika Ijeoma Aniekwu, "Converging Constructions: A Perspective on Sexuality and Feminism in Post-Colonial Africa," *African Sociological Review* 10, no. 1 (2006): 145.
39. Para-Mallam, "Faith, Gender and Development Agendas in Nigeria," 412.

40. See Rosemarie Tong, "The Ethics of Care: A Feminist Virtue Ethics of Care for Healthcare Practitioners," *Journal of Medicine and Philosophy* 23, no. 2 (1998): 141–142.

41. Ibid., 141–142.

42. Thompson, "Conceptualizing Gender in Marriage," 566–567.

43. Abel and Nelson, "Circles of Care," 6.

44. See Fiona Robinson, *The Ethics of Care: A Feminist Approach to Human Security* (Philadelphia, PA: Temple University Press, 2011), 38.

45. Gilligan, "Carol Gilligan."

46. Held, *The Ethics of Care*, 10.

47. Gilligan, "Carol Gilligan."

48. Ibid.

49. Held, *The Ethics of Care*, 135.

50. Ibid.

51. Thompson, "Conceptualizing Gender in Marriage," 566.

52. Also see Tong, "The Ethics of Care," 150.

53. Jane Ribbens McCarthy, "The Powerful Relational Language of 'Family': Togetherness, Belonging and Personhood," *The Sociological Review* 60, no. 1 (2012): 80.

54. "Self-Care Is a Sign of Freedom, Says Michel Foucault," Psychology, *Exploring Your Mind*, last modified November 14, 2017, https://exploringyourmind.com/self-care-sign-freedom-says-michel-foucault/.

55. McCarthy, "The Powerful Relational Language of 'Family'," 70.

Chapter 5

It Is the Fear: Contextualizing the Politics of HIV/AIDS (Non)Disclosure

In this chapter, HIV-seropositive women share their experiences of (non)disclosure and the intense sufferings, emotional pains, and financial hardships that come with it. These are tales that are often untold and sometimes, elided in public health discourses where partner notification also known as HIV status disclosure is touted as an ethical and moral imperative that infected individuals should perform, especially for the overall good of public health. This analysis reveals the complex context-contingent conditions that shape HIV status (non)disclosure among seropositive women in marginalized settings, the ways women rationalize the decisions to disclose or not, and how these decisions produce a set of consequences that women must either navigate or live with.

As we will see, HIV status (non)disclosure, although profoundly configured by social and internalized stigma, is also embedded in the inequalities of gender, social identities, and economic power. As I mentioned in chapter 1 and subsequently reinforced, the household is a traditional and important site of gender analysis mostly because vulnerable female bodies emerge from this space where conflicts in gender, social, and material power coalesce, are expressed, and also contested. In mapping this complex terrain of (non) disclosure, therefore, my focus is mainly on this unit of analysis as well as intimate partner relationships.

Within the broad relations of (non)disclosure, this chapter also attempts to contribute to the existing explanations of female-headed households but through the lens of a new and emerging form of female-headed households that is linked to HIV/AIDS but rarely addressed in the literature. A category of women I refer to as HIV quasi-widows because they do not rigidly fit into the traditional meanings of widowhood in the context of HIV/AIDS, that is, women who have lost their spouses to AIDS. Yet like these women, HIV quasi-widows experience and cope with the social and economic impacts of the virus in isolation but do not receive support like conventional widows.

Quasi-widows are HIV-seropositive women who have been physically or financially abandoned by their spouses. They may or may not live with their spouses but a major underlying characteristic is that they are mostly responsible for the physical and financial responsibilities in their homes because the husbands have shirked their responsibilities.

This concept which I develop throughout the chapter allows us to think about some shortcomings of current modes of interventions that deploy conventional definitions of widowhood and female-heads of households to exclude vulnerable HIV quasi-widows who double as heads of households.

NONDISCLOSURE

As a precursor to women's nondisclosure, identity as intricately linked to social and gender power works in two ways. First, is the notion of *spoiled identities* that is associated with HIV seropositivity.[1] Popular constructions and representations of the pathologies of HIV have been mostly tied to heterosexual relations. With these misperceptions come moral judgments around infected individuals, especially women, who are perceived to have indulged in behaviors that conflict with acceptable cultural and religious norms.

Reduction of stigma around infections and diseases that crisscross sociocultural lines has been linked with drug availability, as such diseases become treatable, and sometimes curable and, thus, gain an unexceptional status.[2] With HIV/AIDS, there has been a reversed reality. Availability of ARTs has not necessarily reduced the social stigma around the infection and disease. And stigma inhibits the uptake of treatment. It also speaks to the exceptionality of HIV/AIDS, which though does not visibly bear identifiable markers of physical deformity but carries with it unparalleled stigma in many spatial contexts where its etiology traverses sociocultural norms and moral lines. In many cases, infected women are socially and morally criminalized, as well as outcast on disclosure of seropositivity due to societal expectations of women as bastions of moral virtues. The protection of identities thus becomes one of the many reasons that knowledge of HIV seropositivity among women is shrouded in secrecy.

In a focus group discussion among HIV-seropositive women—translated from Pidgin English[3] and Urhobo, the latter is one of many local languages in the Niger Delta region—some of the women identified with the misperceptions and stigma around HIV/AIDS, as these have thrust not only their self-image but also their public social identities in tension with societal and moral expectations of womanhood.

HPW 1: What is there to take pride in? [Referring to HIV/AIDS]

HPW 2: You can't talk about it in public.

HPW 1: As a woman who has honor, you can't take pride in it because it is dirty

HPW 2: You can't talk about it.

HPW 3: People will run away from you.

HPW 2: Not everybody says it is caused through needles. They will say you were having indiscriminate sexual relations. And a woman that has indiscriminate sexual relations, what do they call her? They call her a prostitute. This is something that uninfected people do not understand. Although, there are people who still disclose their status. Personally, I can't talk about it [or disclose my status] because the popular opinion is that people get infected through sexual intercourse. It is what most people say, and most of the time, women say this too; women who are illiterate [about HIV] [because] they do not understand.

HPW 4: Prostitution, they would say you got it by sleeping around with other men.

HPW 2: That is why we hide it. . . . We keep it [our status] secret because it is not a good name.

This conversation illuminates the link between spoiled identities and societal constructions of womanhood. HIV seropositivity may imply the affirmation of socially constructed identities and behaviors that are deemed negative and undesired, particularly of married women who are expected to be *faithful and monogamous*, as the conversation indicates. With its associated sexual stigma, HIV seropositivity may not only disrupt desirable identities but also challenge societal concepts of what it is to be *normal* or what it means to be a nondeviant individual.[4]

Stigmatization based on perceived violations of expected norms is not only from men but also from uninfected women as the conversation also indicates. Women who are ignorant about the causalities of HIV perceive that infected women have broken some moral codes and have become an aberration to the essence of womanhood and, thus, confer on such women, spoiled identities. But some HIV-infected women resist these spoiled identities, and one way they do so is through secrecy or nondisclosure especially to uninfected individuals and partners.

A second way that identities work to shape nondisclosure is through social and religious constructions of marriage and motherhood. As established in previous chapters, marriage and motherhood symbolize respect and an increase in social status and, sometimes, improved access to economic capital for many women in Nigeria. Within these structures, women endure hardships and other forms of gender-based violence in order to remain in marital unions than to be socially stigmatized as divorcees or as single mothers. Traditionally, when marriages fail, women are mostly blamed because they are perceived not to have either satisfied their spouses or as irresponsible or did not endure enough even when the men are guilty of wrongdoing. In this social milieu, women are expected to make their marriage work regardless of the circumstance.

> Women are very patient especially when they already have children in the marriage, they don't like leaving their children, they like unity homes but men, any little thing, they are ready to marry ten, six, seven wives but the woman is ready to stay in one place and stay by the children. She is not ready to be bearing [the reputation of having married] three, four, [or] five husbands. See where the problem lies? That is it.—Community health worker

This type of social stigma is one of the reasons why female-heads of households, who are separated from their spouses, although burdened with huge physical and financial responsibilities in catering to themselves and their children, attract less empathy and support from the society, unlike conventional widows.

Women are also reluctant to raise their children without fathers. Rather, they desire to raise their children within the traditional domain of marriage and to maintain the conventional idea of the family. Further narratives revealed that women were more likely to stay with an infected male partner even if they were uninfected but the reverse is the case for an uninfected male spouse and an infected woman. Dissolution of marital unions by men, on the account of seropositivity or other reasons, receives no condemnation because societal norms construct remarriage as typical for men and polygamy as a sign of virility and masculinity.

This also speaks to the culture of dowry or bride price performed by men in many patriarchal African societies like Nigeria, which also enables men to marry as many wives as they choose. The practice of bride price symbolizes male ownership and objectifies women as properties of men, with the bride price considered a sort of marital bond that ties a woman to her husband and his family until it is revoked. Traditionally, a woman is only unbound from her husband and free to remarry when her family has returned the traditional dowry paid on her. However, the divorce rite is a process riddled with shame and stigma for women who decide to go through with it.

For men who decide to remain in union with an infected woman, the family system may maintain the semblance of a traditional family unit but inwardly embody new forms of intra-household dependence and familial relations as power relations are intensified. Family dynamics may be reconfigured such that existing hierarchies within the household are reinforced in ways that the already-subservient female partner becomes even more powerless.

For an HIV-infected woman, disclosure of seropositivity to whom she may consider an uninfected spouse may mean that she may lose her marriage and her home, especially by a partner who may be unwilling to support her. Such women tend not to disclose their seropositivity. Interestingly, she never gets to find out if her partner is also seropositive and if he was the source of her infection, unless the man discloses as well. In instances where some of these women found out their husband's seropositivity, it was at the level of full-blown AIDS or when the spouse's death was confirmed to be from AIDS. It was at this point these women sought to get tested and were diagnosed like their spouses, to be HIV positive.

Nondisclosure is a strong correlate for lack of treatment initiation and in situations when HIV treatment is initiated, adherence can become very problematic.

> There is another case of a lady that is positive but the husband is negative and the husband did not know she was positive, and she being scared that she does not want to lose her marriage, does not come to access her drugs. She is on her own because she does not access her drugs.—HIV-seropositive woman and support group leader

For the youngest participant in the focus group discussions, a woman who appeared to be in her early to mid-twenties, marriage has been expectedly a major concern. It is common knowledge and experience among this group that seropositivity greatly diminishes the opportunities for marriage. With a previously failed relationship due to disclosure of her seropositivity, her fears are further justified and hence her resolution to not disclose her status to her current partner. According to her:

> What about me, how do I get married? I am afraid. . . . This is the reason why I won't tell him because the first man [I told], he already knew my situation and that is why he ran away from me. It is the fear that if I tell my current boyfriend that he will leave me just as the previous one [did], which is why there is no need to tell him. . . . Why do I not take my drugs? It is because I am living with my boyfriend so the day he is at home, I won't take it that day. When he goes to work, I will take the drugs. I do not want to disclose to him.—HIV-seropositive woman

This excerpt also reveals the dilemma women face in treatment adherence. In cases of nondisclosure, women adopt strategies to continue the secrecy of their seropositivity even as they access treatment but to the detriment of adherence. Still, this narrative provides insights into one of the many reasons that shape women's disposition to not disclose their seropositivity. Women who had experienced discrimination and rejection through partner or spousal abandonment after disclosure in previous relationships appeared to be less poised to disclose to new partners. Similarly, another HIV-seropositive woman, but this time in a marital relationship, who had experienced rejection and abandonment, narrates her ordeal, in this translated excerpt.

> He asked me to pack my things and leave the house but because I refused to pack, he packed and left me. So the children and I remained in the house. Later on, he said he will not continue to pay for the house rent so I had to pack and leave the house to a cheaper place. It is in this cheap place that the children and I are living now. He does not even care for the children. I am the only who does. It is the farming that I do that I use in taking care of these children, to pay their school fees. . . . If the man I had children for abandoned me when I disclosed my status to him, why will another person whom I do not even have such connections to not do the same? I will not disclose. Even if I am dying here, even if HIV/AIDS is what is killing me, I will not disclose. And if at all I remarry, I will never disclose my status.—HIV-seropositive woman

Based on the narratives, the rationalization to disclose or not to disclose is permeated through the politics of everyday life within and outside intimate partner relations. Psychosocially, the process of disclosure or nondisclosure involves a personal cognitive evaluation of the status of intimate, marital, and social relationships, where women assess if their male partner or others love them enough to accept their status or reject them on disclosure. Such evaluations are performed in the context of real and perceived risks associated with the process of disclosure whether as personally experienced in previous relationships or by the experiences of others. It also means that there must be a perceived level of trust in intimate partner relations that either determines or motivates women to disclose or not—the nature of relationships matters as some of the women claimed.

Disclosure, thus, comes with trust and feelings of personal security as some of the women claimed that perceptions of the degree of love of a partner toward a woman also help to guide her decision-making process. This was the case of the few women in this group who had disclosed their seropositivity to their spouses. Among the twenty-two HIV-seropositive women interviewed for this study, only three had disclosed their seropositivity to their male partners and were still living with their spouses at the time of the discussions.

Also important to note is that two of these three seropositive women were educated, and the other was a small business owner. I mention this to highlight the possibility that their socioeconomic status may have played some role in their disclosure. Although I did not immediately pursue this line of inquiry, their narratives indicated that like other women, they struggled with their decisions to disclose. In addition to perceived levels of trust in their relationships, and knowledge received from HIV counseling, they felt a personal sense of moral duty to inform their partners of their status.

Interestingly, two of these three women on disclosure found out that their male partners were also positive and were the sources of their infections. The third woman whose husband was uninfected and who had lost a baby to AIDS—which is the way she found out that she was HIV positive—was later determined to have been infected by a traditional birth attendant during child delivery. However, only two of the three women claimed to have received consistent support from their spouses after disclosure. Also, two of these three women have gone on to become the leaders of the HIV support group at the health facility, following up and monitoring members' adherence to treatment, as well as helping other women in the disclosure process. Despite their experiences of disclosure, these HIV-seropositive women and support group leaders maintain that most infected women do not disclose to their husbands or partners especially when the assessed risks outweigh the perceived benefits, with some of these benefits being emotional, social, and financial support.

> There was the case of a lady, she is the second wife of the husband, and the husband came to [marry] her because the [first] wife at home cannot produce a child. [So] she was the one doing the production of kids for the man [but] she is [HIV] positive. So when I asked her to disclose, she said she won't try it that the husband is going to run away and abandon the kids for her.—HIV-seropositive woman and support group leader

The practice of disclosure often comes at a personal price and one that many HIV-seropositive women are unwilling to pay. Women generally feel that because of their marginalized status, it is easier for them to lose their relationships, homes, social securities, and identities, whether as single or married women on disclosure. Fear of rejection and spousal abandonment especially where kids are involved and being solely saddled with the social and financial responsibilities associated with child upbringing, threats of domestic violence, and inability to attract a potential spouse for marriage, were the commonly cited reasons for nondisclosure.

These narratives also expose the materiality and economic rationalizations that underpin the process of disclosure. Power distribution between partners, for example, who controls the economic decision making process for resource allocation, is also a crucial factor in rationalizing the decision to disclose. Directly or indirectly, this dynamic shapes treatment uptake and adherence. Nevertheless, these individualized assessments of risks are actually a microcosm of broader social and economic arrangements that adversely interact with women on a very personal level in ways that render them powerless. This structural dimension of nondisclosure is one that is obscured in the HIV/

AIDS discourse yet it is significant to fully grasping the range of factors that constrict nondisclosure. Consequently, interventions aimed at facilitating and improving disclosure at the level of the individual are less effective because they ignore the connections that the body makes with structural forces as well as the associated negative impacts.

Coming to terms with such structural forces destabilizes conventional notions of individual agency and choice that are common in traditional HIV/AIDS discourse wherein women are positioned as freely capable of making the decision to disclose or not. These forces, although hidden, work in complex ways through the private lives of women such that they are rarely addressed in mainstream research and interventions. Disclosure is, thus, never an objective or neutral process or practice as it is sometimes conceived in theory—a simple and homogenous process that produces uniform outcomes for all who practice it.

Counseling is a common practice deployed to engender HIV-status disclosure post-diagnosis in Nigerian healthcare settings. It is also aimed at reworking the fears and insecurities of the disclosing individual. Sometimes, this process includes pre-disclosure counseling of the other partner to elicit a positive reaction in the event of disclosure. When partner notification is successful, post-disclosure counseling is thus extended to both partners, and sometimes with recommendation for testing, especially when the partners disclosed to may be unaware of their status. While this practice has shown some positive impacts, it is yet another individualized strategy that subordinates women's fate to the whims and decisions of their male partners, as demonstrated by cases where women with little-to-no socioeconomic leverage suffer both seropositivity and abandonment. Partner notification as espoused by existing global guidelines can, thus, potentially become a double-edged sword, in the sense that the individuals suffer while the public benefits. This is particularly so in spatial contexts where less attention is paid to the conditions in which disclosure takes place or under circumstances considered as being in the "best interests of the individual."[5]

International guidelines on disclosure by World Health Organization (WHO) and the United Nations Agency for the Control of AIDS (UNAIDS), which appear to be rarely followed in local healthcare contexts, stipulate as follows:

> Provider-initiated HIV testing and counseling efforts must be made to ensure that a supportive social, policy and legal framework is in place to maximize positive outcomes and minimize potential harms to patients. Adaptation of this guidance at country level will require an assessment of the local epidemiology as well as the risks and benefits of provider-initiated HIV testing and counseling, including an appraisal of available resources, prevailing standards of HIV prevention, treatment, care and support, and the adequacy of social and

> legal protections available. . . . Service providers should always aim to do what is best in the best interests of the individual patient. Endorsements of provider-initiated HIV testing and counseling by WHO and UNAIDS is not an endorsement of coercive or mandatory HIV testing. WHO and UNAIDS do not support mandatory or compulsory testing of individuals on public health grounds.[6]

In the present context, however, not all or most of these conditions are present during the process of counseling and testing initiated by health service providers. There is rarely a sociolegal framework to act as a buffer especially against the harmful outcomes of disclosure, as the following quotes indicate:

> We try to counsel them; that is what we do. We try to counsel them and we leave them to their fate.—Community healthcare worker

> I encourage women to disclose . . . because when the virus gets serious and you fall very sick, that man that you are hiding your status from, you won't even know when you will disclose your status to him especially when things get worse. So the best thing is to open up to him now so that he just knows, and if he wants to abandon you, let him abandon you, provided you have done your part by opening up to him.—[Translated] HIV-seropositive woman and support group leader

In local healthcare settings, focus appears to be more on the mandate to persuade individuals to disclose and less concern about anticipated outcomes. While it may seem empowering for women to disclose their status, the outcomes may be disempowering for some. Yet, through the counseling process, where infected individuals are reminded of their moral responsibilities to their partners, these individuals might feel pressured to disclose. Similarly, in the steps preceding disclosure like testing, some health workers have reported instances of pregnant women seeking antenatal care who were tested for HIV but were not preinformed and neither were their consent sought for fear that they will refuse to be tested. Although this is unethical within the practice of medicine and as the WHO guideline above shows, this behavior was rationalized as the need to protect incoming generations from the disease irrespective of patients' informed consent, as doing otherwise would mean an increase in mother-to-child transmission.

In a society where women are more likely to remain in abusive relationships because of fear of losing their social and economic protection, partner counseling as the only strategy to enable safe disclosure leaves women with fewer choices to deal with negative outcomes. The reported abuse women suffer from their male partners on disclosure calls to question if there are existing strategies on handling the negative outcomes of disclosure among this already vulnerable and marginalized population. How these women are assisted to move forward and psychologically reoriented to enable future disclosure despite previous negative experiences such that continued HIV transmission can be halted should form a crucial component of HIV/AIDS programming.

But as common practices at the Erhoike health center (and many other centers across the country) show, disclosure strategies are more directed at actual disclosure but less on addressing potential and actual social, psychological, and material outcomes that confront women when this process goes awry. This is not because of any fault of the health centers but because the resources to do so are not provided by the relevant institutions. To this end, many of the HIV-seropositive women expressed a range of emotions from regret, self-pity, anger, and bitterness because of their seropositivity as they claimed emotional, social, and financial isolation within and outside their intimate relationships.

In the next section, I shed light on the most commonly cited consequences of disclosure, which are spousal rejection and abandonment, and the ways these are disrupting the dynamics of intimate relationships and gradually changing the traditional family structure. From a policy standpoint, I look at how HIV quasi-widows even as vulnerable subjects are overlooked in interventions through rigid designations of widowhood and contextual framings of female-headed households as well as the implications for treatment access and adherence.

HIV/AIDS AND THE CHANGING FAMILY STRUCTURE: QUASI-WIDOWHOOD

One of the psychosocial implications of HIV/AIDS in the relevant scholarship includes the reconfiguration of the family system and the changing gender roles within it.[7] In past studies, changes in family structures from HIV/AIDS have been mostly conceived in terms of household composition, shifts in gender roles, and dependency burden.[8] If the male spouse, usually the head of the home, is the one infected by the disease, his bodily incapacitation may necessitate the female partner taking on a headship role especially from an economic viewpoint, if she has the ability. The provider status is thus swapped as the woman doubles as the primary breadwinner and caregiver. In some spatial contexts, the decision-making structure and process may be reconfigured as a shift in economic power may translate to decision-making power and privilege for women. These are the classic documentation of the disease's impact on the restructuring of the conventional nuclear family system that comprises immediate kinships of filial and parental relations.[9] In other words, mortality to HIV/AIDS may produce change in provider status of the traditional male-heads and thus culminate in the formation of female-heads or single-parent households.[10]

In contrast, however, the impact of HIV status disclosure on marital and social arrangements, although well documented, is less addressed as a problematic development to the structure of conventional families and social systems, in general. In particular, the link between HIV/AIDS disclosure and the formation and rise of HIV female-headed households, or more specifically, a typology that this study designates as HIV quasi-widows because of the unique role that seropositivity plays in this formation, is obscured. I distinguish between two forms of HIV quasi-widows: those who live separately from their spouses and those who live with their spouses.

Many HIV-seropositive women lamented the absence of their husbands and intimate partners from rejection and abandonment due to the disclosure of their seropositivity. HIV quasi-widows are the products of absentee or runaway husbands. Absentee husbands include men who may not or still be legally married to their wives but may have physically or financially checked out of their spousal and paternal obligations. HIV-seropositive women from either monogamous, polygamous or informal consensual unions, who are rejected and abandoned by their partners post disclosure of seropositivity, may be separated or divorced and operate as single parents or heads of households with the children from such unions. This category of HIV quasi-widows may live on their own because of divorce or separation.

The second category of HIV quasi-widows is seropositive women who live with their male partners or spouses, in both formal and informal unions but are also the main income providers or heads of their households because they receive little or no spousal support. Sometimes, seropositivity may not be solely at fault for male irresponsibility especially where the woman's seropositivity is undisclosed. However, the underlying premise is that HIV-seropositive women's vulnerabilities are increased when they are in spousal unions but mostly bear the physical and financial burden of caring for their families.

In the Niger Delta region, in general, spousal irresponsibility is also a function of the existing social ethos which fosters irresponsibility among men who are not educated or oriented into appropriate forms of masculinity such that they shirk their financial, social, and physical responsibilities to their wives and children, even for women who are not seropositive. In cases of multiple or separate households where the woman may be living alone with the children, the male partner or husband may, however, show up at will to claim his conjugal rights even when he provides no financial support to the household. Also complicating the narrative of absentee husbands that has aided demographic shifts in the creation of single female-parent households in the Niger Delta is the social impacts of oil degradation in the region that compel men to relocate from agrarian geographies to the cities to seek alternative means of livelihoods, following the destruction of their ecological environment and traditional means of occupation, leaving behind children and wives for long periods and sometimes, permanently.[11]

In both types of HIV quasi-widowhood, affected women fit into the formal convention of female-headed households, defined by the International Labor Organization as:

> households where either no adult males are present, owing to divorce, separation, migration, non-marriage or widowhood; *or where the men, although present, do not contribute to the household income* because of illness or disability, old age, alcoholism or similar incapacity (but not because of unemployment). [Emphasis mine][12]

In other definitions, a female-headed household is that "in which an adult female is the sole or main income producer and *decision-maker* [Emphasis mine]."[13] The emphasis in the preceding definition is to establish a contrast with local conventions of female-headed households in the present cultural milieu. In Nigeria, households where a male spouse is physically present but a woman is the primary economic provider or makes financial contributions equal to or greater than the man, women in such instances are usually not considered as the heads of the household or decision-makers because patriarchal social customs confer headship of households to men whether they live up to their provider status or not. The power of decision-making may be true for female-heads of households who are living alone but depending on specific relationships, men may still wield some sort of control especially over decisions that relate to the children even with separation or divorce.

I discuss, subsequently in this chapter, the policy implication of the local characterization of heads of households in this spatial context for HIV-seropositive women. Qualitative evidence that emerged from this study also proffers additional insight into the growing trend of female-headed households and absentee husbands in Nigeria,[14] and illuminates a new demographic shift in the traditional family configuration, which is the creation of HIV quasi-widows in HIV/AIDS-affected regions like the Niger Delta.

An interesting paradox that emerged from the women's narratives is that while women preferred to remain in union with their spouses and partners, their physical presence was reported to inhibit access and adherence especially in situations where women had not disclosed their status, and therefore, were unable to adequately sustain treatment uptake for fear of exposure. In this sense, treatment uptake was done in secrecy when the spouse or partner was physically unavailable. On the other hand, absentee husbands were also cited as a barrier to access and adherence to treatment due to the lack of economic security that marital relationships are expected to yield because of the dominant identity of men are as providers, as have been reiterated throughout this book. HIV quasi-widows, thus, suffer treatment challenges due to spousal abandonment as the following scenario depicts.

> Most of them that you are seeing [HIV-seropositive women] stopped to take their treatment due to not being able to provide for themselves, in terms of their husbands running away after disclosing their status. So they have not been able to provide for themselves in terms of how to care for their own personal needs and there is no way they can take the drugs like that without something to eat especially where there is no work for them to do. They don't have work to do. They don't even know how to go about most of their own personal activities and some, [these are] some of the problems we encounter here as the executives of the support group. You see some [of these women], they complain to you in terms of their home rentage, [that is] how to pay their rent, they don't really have that, they don't have it [the financial resources]. Then some [of the women], after losing their husbands, they don't even know how to go about anything anymore.—HIV-seropositive woman and support group leader

HIV-seropositive women who are abandoned and live separately with their kids are suddenly thrust to become heads of their households, yet they are disempowered. Although this may shift the balance of power toward them in decision-making, they are pushed further down the ladder of poverty and economic vulnerability as the excerpt above demonstrates. In patriarchal societies where public and economic spaces are mostly dominated and regarded as the enterprise of men, HIV-seropositive women as heads of households and providers are doubly challenged to compete with other men for available economic opportunities, and with little to no education or skills, their economic options are further diminished. Socially, women as heads of household who live alone, although may now have some autonomy, embody a spoiled identity because of the perceived stigma attached to women with children but without husbands due to separation or divorce. Hence, some women decide to remain quasi-widows within marital households with physically present spouses in order to disconnect from the stigma of a spoiled identity and other negative social impacts on the family unit.

Impacts of the dislocation of the family unit transcend the couple as children become unwilling casualties in such spaces. Sometimes, children as products of broken homes drop out of school to share the breadwinning responsibilities when their mothers are unable meet up with the financial obligations of the household, thereby, increasing their risks and vulnerabilities. By implication, this reconfigured version of the family system although expands the population of HIV vulnerable subjects, they are often outside the radar of formal and informal interventions that prioritize conventional widows for particular social and financial services where available. Reason is that both categories of quasi-widows do not neatly fall within the traditional definitions of HIV/AIDS widows either because of existing marital connections or because the absence of husbands is not due to death. Yet these are infected women who need care for themselves but remain burdened with providing care for their households as they grapple with impoverished and austere conditions. Similarly, female-heads of households, whether from HIV/AIDS or otherwise, do not receive the same level of empathy from the society as conventional widows do; rather, they are stigmatized.

In much of sub-Saharan Africa, the family is traditionally considered a strong safety net of social support and material stability.[15] This may also be true for other geographies. HIV/AIDS international guidelines designate vulnerable households to include those with one or both infected partners[16] as well as vulnerable children—children within infected households and children orphaned by HIV/AIDS—with existing interventions for HIV-affected children like the orphans and vulnerable children programs.[17]

For adults, however, welfare and empowerment programs such as cash transfers and skills acquisition appear to be more focused on traditional widows or households that have experienced death of a parent to AIDS. Widows from such unions have become a focal population because they fall within the official definition of widowhood.[18] Although not aptly defined, the operationalization of the term, "widows" by the United Nations Women and other international organizations show conventional forms of usage as women who have lost their spouses to mortality.[19] HIV quasi-widows are thus less visible because they do not clearly cut the picture of the traditional vulnerable widows and female-heads of households and, thus, may only be able to access available empowerment programs based on some other criteria.

HIV quasi-widows who are physically present with their spouses fall through the cracks of interventions that may be otherwise accessible to traditional widows because their marital identities which are perceived conditions for social and economic security veil their true vulnerabilities. Furthermore, HIV quasi-widows whether they live alone or not are also disadvantaged in the same way because of local characterizations of female-headed households that fall below the conventional standards—a shortcoming in the Nigerian context that shows a biased understanding of what truly constitutes female-headed households.

Disclosure as a process can be empowering for public health goals, yet inimical to women's welfare. Undoubtedly, HIV/AIDS disclosure may embody dire and unwanted consequences for already-marginalized individuals who are less able to tackle the effects of this disease, especially in settings where social and welfare services are inadequate or inherently lacking. And women disproportionately fall within this marginal population. HIV-seropositive women's experiences and narratives illuminate a gap in interventions, which is the lack of social workers and psychotherapists, and when available, their inadequacy to ameliorate some of the burden of seropositivity. HIV-seropositive women do not only deal with the material conditions of their status but they also have to deal with the emotional and psychosocial impacts, especially in situations where their disclosure disrupts their normal social functions and intimate networks. But there is little around psychosocial coping strategies for women to reduce such stressors as local health workers double to function in this role but inadequately so.

Women's narratives of the barriers to treatment access and adherence are proof that addressing negative intra-household shifts and dynamics will greatly enhance uptake and adherence to treatment. To facilitate access and adherence to treatment among this population, micro-level interventions must also be restructured to focus on the family through theoretical research of a psychosocial nature and policies that focus on the personal and intimate forces that may affect care. It begins by reconceptualizing the HIV-seropositive woman, first as a social being and second, as part of the larger constituency of the family unit.

It is important to note that traditionally, HIV/AIDS interventions have addressed the nuclear family as a household unit especially in the practice of counseling serodiscordant couples prior to testing, diagnosis, and disclosure. HIV/AIDS programs targeted at the family or household unit are, however, mostly limited to the infected individuals. The long-term undesirable social and material effects of disclosure on general household dynamics that also include the vulnerability of children are often neglected. Nevertheless, the practice of couples counseling is evidence of the growing recognition of the household, especially the nuclear family unit, as an important scale of intervention but one that needs to be far-reaching and holistic to include other psychosocial and material implications.

Not only it is important that the household, in its broader dimensions, is considered a scale of intervention, but it is also important that local definitions of widows and female-headed households, especially in the context of HIV/AIDS interventions, are displaced and redefined such that policies also contemplate and address the vulnerability of HIV quasi-widows as female-heads of households, whether physically present in a marital union or not.

NOTES

1. See Erving Goffman, *Stigma: Notes on the Management of Spoiled Identity* (Englewood Cliffs, NJ: Prentice Hall, 1963).

2. Lisanne Brown, Lea Trujillo, and Kate Macintyre, *Interventions to Reduce HIV/AIDS Stigma: What Have We Learned?* (New Orleans: The Population Council, 2001), 15.

3. The Nigerian Pidgin English is an informal English-based creole language with origins from the Portuguese slave trade era, which is spoken as a *lingua franca* (in addition to the Standard English) across Nigeria, with variations found in Cameroun, Ghana, and some other parts of West Africa.

4. Frye et al., "Managing Identity Impacts Associated with Disclosure of HIV Status: A Qualitative Investigation," *AIDS Care: Psychological and Socio-Medical Aspects of AIDS/HIV* 21, no. 8 (2009): 1072, https://doi.org/10.1080/09540120802657514.

5. World Health Organization and Joint United Nations Program on HIV/AIDS, *Guidance on Provider-Initiated HIV Testing and Counselling in Health Facilities* (Geneva: World Health Organization and Joint United Nations Program on HIV/AIDS, 2007), 6, https://www.who.int/hiv/pub/guidelines/9789241595568_en.pdf.

6. Ibid., 5–6.

7. James P. M. Ntozi and Samuel Zirimenya, "Changes in Household Composition and Family Structure during the AIDS Epidemic in Uganda," *The Continuing African HIV/AIDS Epidemic* (1999): 194; Robert Bor, Riva Miller, and Eleanor Goldman, "HIV/AIDS and the Family: A Review of Research in the First Decade," *Journal of Family Therapy* 15 (1993): 188–189.

8. See findings from studies like Ntozi and Zirimenya, "Changes in Household Composition and Family Structure"; Erick Otieno Nyambedha, Simiyu Wandibba, and Jens Aagaard-Hansen, "Changing Patterns of Orphan Care Due to the HIV Epidemic in Western Kenya," *Social Science and Medicine* 57 (2003); Bor, Miller, and Goldman, "HIV/AIDS and the Family."

9. Ibid.

10. Ntozi and Zirimenya, "Changes in Household Composition and Family Structure," 194.

11. Emem Bassey Iyang and Ekaete Evans Udong, "Livelihood Insecurity and Diversification among Women in an Environmentally Challenged Niger Delta Region, Nigeria," *The International Journal of Humanities and Social Science* 1, no. 1 (2013): 44. Also see Eno Okoko, "Women and Environmental Change in the Niger Delta, Nigeria: Evidence from Ibeno," *Gender Place and Culture* 6, no. 4 (1999): 375–376, https://doi.org/10.1080/09663699924944.

12. International Labor Organization, *ABC of Women Workers' Rights and Gender Equality* (Geneva: International Labor Organization, 2007), 81, https://www.ilo.org/wcmsp5/groups/public/---dgreports/---gender/documents/publication/wcms_087314.pdf.

13. "Female-headed Households," Gender Equality Glossary and Thesaurus, European Institute for Gender Equality, accessed February 9, 2019, https://eige.europa.eu/rdc/thesaurus/terms/1126.

14. See Felicia Durojaiye Oyekanmi, "Institutionalization of Gender Inequality in Nigeria: Implications for the Advancement of Women," *Population Review* 44, no. 1 (2005), https://doi.org/10.1353/prv.2005.0005, for explanations on the growing trend of female-headed households in Nigeria but mainly attributed to increasing female empowerment.

15. Floyd et al., "The Long Term Social and Economic Impact of HIV on the Spouses of Infected Individuals in Northern Malawi," *Tropical Medicine and International Health* 13, no. 4 (2008): 529, doi:10.1111/j.1365–3156.2008.02030.x.

16. United Nations World Food Program (WFP), *HIV/AIDS Analysis: Integrating HIV/AIDS in Food Security and Vulnerability Analysis* (Rome: Vulnerability Analysis and Mapping Branch and HIV/AIDS Service, 2008), 23, https://documents.wfp.org/stellent/groups/public/documents/manual_guide_proced/wfp193482.pdf.

17. Ibid., 28, 53.

18. "International Widow's Day, 23 June," United Nations, accessed September 14, 2018, http://www.un.org/en/events/widowsday/. Also see "Statement: Widows Rights to Independent Life and Livelihood after Loss," United Nations Women, last modified June 21, 2017, http://www.unwomen.org/en/news/stories/2017/6/statement-un-women-international-widows-day.

19. For example, see United Nations, *Widowhood: Invisible, Secluded or Excluded* (Geneva: United Nations Division for the Advancement of Women, 2001), http://www.un.org/womenwatch/daw/public/wom_Dec%2001%20single%20pg.pdf.

Chapter 6

Feminism and the Conflicting Discourses of Empowerment

> *Feminism. You know how we feel about that embarrassing Western philosophy? The destroyer of homes. Imported mainly from America to ruin nice African homes.*
>
> —Aidoo (1989)[1]

This chapter furthers the discourse on the feminized pattern of ARV access and adherence but at the intersection of women's social and material disempowerment, as well as the corresponding local discourses of empowerment that are shaped by culture, gendered identities, and need for social security, within the context of patriarchy. Again, the debates and claims in this chapter are made through the lens of women at the grassroots, who are also HIV-seropositive.

First, this chapter uncovers local but unorthodox discourses of empowerment—unorthodox because they do not fit popular or universal notions—in an attempt to diversify the ways that we imagine women's empowerment in development scholarship and practice. Second, the chapter deploys practical evidence to assert the notion that empowerment like many social concepts is fluid, culturally contingent, and experienced in a range of ways that also border on individual social, economic, and class locations. And third, based on the centrality of the concept of women's empowerment to the gender equality and feminist agenda, this chapter also shows the different ways that cultural discourses on empowerment among HIV-seropositive women complicate stereotypical Western ideologies on feminism and indigenous feminism as practiced in the Nigerian context. At this juncture, I also argue that indigenous feminism in this context is not inclusive of all dimensions of women's lived experiences or reflective of the diversity of gendered worldviews that exist in this geography. I engage with these perspectives as they emanated from the qualitative data, especially in terms of the ways that feminist activists and development practitioners might effectively engage local discourses of empowerment even when these are in conflict with the mainstream.

Traditional critiques of mainstream Eurocentric notions of development projects purported for the Global South have argued against the re-perpetuation of the Global South's dependence on the Global North as Western development projects enervate the South's abilities to make autonomous choices and map out its own development trajectory.[2] This trend of power and hierarchies in development thought and practice, broadly, is one that, I argue, is reproduced at a much local scale.

The term disempowerment, although cuts across gender groups, is mostly conflated with women in gender development policy and practice, especially women of low socioeconomic status.[3] Thus, women with access to some level of power and privilege have been mostly involved in the struggles of emancipation and empowerment for women of lower status. Advocacy for female emancipation by powerful interest groups that take up the fight for other less powerful women is, however, usually based on values and assumptions perceived to be beneficial to the subjects' interests. It becomes imperative to not only understand how poor women as mostly targets and beneficiaries of empowerment programs, utilize and appropriate the concept of empowerment but also the ways that it is interpreted and pushed for by women advocates and feminist groups.

Likewise, existing tensions in modern feminist discourses have involved contestations on the universalization of Western feminism to all spatial contexts like the third world, irrespective of disparities in the historical, modern, political, cultural, social, and religious contexts that shape the relations of gender power in these places.[4] Nevertheless, global contentions on diversity and difference, and the struggle to eliminate these disparities in both feminist scholarship and practice should not in any way suggest that the feminist movement is homogenous even within third world spaces. Based on the evidence that has emerged from this research, new forms of representational politics in feminist scholarship and practice are continually reproduced within national and subnational contexts, with social and class differences implicated in the disparate ways that feminism is imagined and mapped out by indigenous feminist movements in Nigeria.

My intention is not to run a commentary on feminism in Nigeria but to deconstruct particular ideologies pushed forward by indigenous feminist organizations, for example, the Nigerian Feminist Forum (NFF) which appears to be at the forefront of the feminist movement in Nigeria, and the ways that their ideologies traverse discourses of empowerment at the grassroots, especially among HIV-seropositive women. And how, if there are any ideological conflicts, the ways that these may illuminate our understanding of why local empowerment programs for women at the grassroots, especially among poor women, meet with so much resistance and fail to achieve their intended objectives. Also significant to the choice of these indigenous feminist organizations as a reference to highlight local discourses of empowerment in this context, is the need to understand how the notion of empowerment becomes fluid across a seemingly monolithic group, in this case women, especially when intersected with other axes of social difference besides gender. This is particularly so because the experiences of HIV-seropositive women show that their social locations and demographics made considerable impact on how they experienced the disease as well as associated interventions like treatment.

Also apparent in women's testimonies is how these multiple axes of their marginality—as uneducated, underprivileged, and poor women, many of whom are confined to agrarian spaces with livelihoods that have become unsustainable over time due to environmental challenges—have not only structured the nature of their needs but also corresponding discourses of empowerment, as we will see later in this chapter. While geography and culture provided broad influences in the ways these women imagined empowerment, this analysis narrows down to how feminism or the struggle for female emancipation may also be influenced by individual attributes like class and socioeconomic power, thereby, contributing to popular analyses of feminism that are from purely geographical and cultural perspectives.[5] In this way, this chapter foregrounds the dynamism of women's engagement with gender relations in the Nigerian context and contributes to indigenous discourses of female empowerment but as have emerged from women at the grassroots.[6]

Gender is not experienced in homogenous ways—a conception that has given materiality to the diversity and fluidity of gender as a construct. Gender variabilities are also symbolic of the centrality of biology, sexual orientation, and social and economic factors as they produce unique individual needs as well as diverse gendered experiences, even within groups of women or men. Arguably, while there might be great commonalities and shared interests, for example, in the needs of women within particular spatial contexts, gendered needs are unstable and changing, especially at the intersection of other axes of social difference, in time and place. It makes sense, therefore, to explore probable areas of disconnect and convergence in the feminist agenda between women as activists and women as subjects of empowerment, and how the intersections of class, socioeconomic power, and privilege may affect the diverse ways that the gender equality agenda is imagined and referenced by women in the Nigerian context.

What may be regarded as feminist scholarship in Nigeria is dominated by female literary writers and critics who through their stories focused on everyday encounters of women in Nigeria's patriarchal context, and many of whom refused to identify as feminists but over time, some have come to embrace the feminist label.[7] But the challenge of theorizing an all-inclusive feminism that encompasses the diversity of women's experiences and divergent gendered ideologies is expressed in the different variants of feminism that have emerged in Nigeria over time, from motherism, womanism, stiwanism, nego-feminism to snail-sense feminism but all cater to a distinct experience of the Nigerian woman—her encounter with patriarchy.[8] I provide a brief summary of these variants.[9]

Motherism celebrates rural women as nurturers of society on the basis of their productive roles as food producers through farming, in confrontation with the modern urban woman who contemporary society regards in higher esteem given her education, economic independence, and general assertiveness. Motherism deems the urban woman devoid of the virtue of nurture—in this case, to society through a relationship with land and nature. Womanism, which is an intercontinental variant, foregrounds a confrontation with culture, colonialism, and other types of domination that have oppressed the continental and diasporic black African woman. Stiwanism, on the other hand, narrows feminism more geographically to the issues of women living in Africa and in the African context. Nego-feminism and snail-sense feminism are rooted in the idea of inclusion, complementarity, and collaboration with men based on the knowledge of local cultural systems and thus, the idea of diplomacy, negotiation, and nonconfrontation with patriarchy.

Also common to these indigenous feminist models is the connection to culture, religion, heterosexuality, and a resistance to Western feminism, for example, a rejection of gay politics and the exclusion of men from feminist spaces.[10] Nevertheless, the Nigerian feminist landscape seems to be evolving especially with more recent feminist organizations like the NFF which advances a radical approach to feminism with ideals that are antithetical to these earlier models of feminism, particularly the latter's total rejection of Western feminism. Perhaps, the fluidity of gender and its diverse experiences according to time and place, as well as the socioreligious locations of individuals are complicit in the plethora of discourses and variants of feminism in Nigeria, which also made it impossible for me to find a coherent body of knowledge that succinctly depicts what Nigerian feminism is. Rather, I found excerpts of philosophical thoughts and ideologies which are mostly situated within the broader African feminist discourse that also critiqued strands of feminism that originated from the West. At the time of writing this book, there is still not an absolute or coherent discourse on Nigerian feminism but what I present here, which forms most of the analytical base for this chapter, are feminist ideologies from the most prominent feminist movement in Nigeria, the NFF.

Established in 2008, the NFF is the first women's movement in Nigeria to formally identify with the global feminist movement in form and principle through oral and written texts. It is also remarkably different from other national or local women's movements from historical to present time in Nigeria, given its aggressive and radical stance, as well as embrace of Western feminist ideals; hence, it is crucial to this analysis, especially because it brings a view of feminism that is not typical in this context.

CLARIFYING AND CONTEXTUALIZING EMPOWERMENT THROUGH LOCAL VOICES

The term empowerment is loaded; thus, any attempt to ascribe a mainstream definition will fall short of being holistic and representative of its multiple dimensions. Hence, my task in this section is to illuminate some of its varied dimensions and place these in context. At its core, however, empowerment simply means to grant an individual power and ability to do something. Beyond *giving power and ability* is also the idea of empowerment as an agency that makes it possible for individuals to act self-confidently in controlling their lives and advocating for their rights. Empowerment, thus, connotes a preexisting state of disempowerment that is embedded in the powerlessness and vulnerability of marginalized subjects. As it relates to women, disempowerment implies that women lack power in whatever forms that it (power) is available, whether material or incorporeal, which also signifies the need for equity.

Within a gendered framework, empowerment discourses also involve the discursive formations of women's disempowerment and the context in which these are produced, whether as a function of power imbalance, inequalities, or social hierarchies. Central to the concept of empowerment, therefore, is power.[11] Power is what sustains hierarchies and it is inextricably linked to empowerment (and disempowerment), and synonymous with whether a subject is equipped or not with the ability (power) to do something. In this sense, power can be oppressive and may embody conflict where one group is conscious of its subordination or domination with respect to group or individual interests.[12]

Universal concepts of female empowerment rooted in Western philosophy have traditionally been constructed in material terms taking the form of financial empowerment, but in time, they shifted to include empowerment through formal education and rights to participate in political life.[13] While such forms of empowerment have been theorized in the women in development (WID) literature as enhancing decision-making in the household, the imbalance in gender power remains uninfluenced and unchanged, especially in patriarchal contexts. An explanation for this is that empowerment in this context is premised on the norms and values of patriarchy, and which appear non-negotiable because they are deeply entrenched at all levels of life and social reproduction.

This also speaks to the mutability of empowerment and compels us to ask context-specific questions in order to understand its situatedness as a function of specific geographies even as we take into account its more global connections. This is not a sequential order in which the word empowerment is imagined but this reasoning frames the multilayers and broad dimensions from which I approach (dis)empowerment.

Generally, empowerment in mainstream development has been deployed in uncritically universal ways to exclude local variants and discourses of empowerment. HIV-seropositive women, in this context, sought forms of empowerment that can translate to economic and material power in ways that increase their bargaining and negotiating power within intimate and household relations but not necessarily empowerment as a social emancipation from male control and domination. For example, lack of access and adherence to treatment were mainly attributed to a lack of economic empowerment due to absentee husbands and also their own personal disempowerment. Women appeared either oblivious to the paradox of their reality in that their current vulnerabilities are the products of patriarchal structures which sustain current forms of hierarchies such that their economic security is intricately linked to the presence or absence of men in their lives. Or perhaps, there is a silent acceptance of unequal conditions by women in the perceived absence of real alternatives.

Women, thus, constructed empowerment in a narrow form that is limited to material empowerment through employment and sustainable livelihoods such that they can cater to their own needs—a departure from formal feminist discourses of female liberation that encompass social, religious, political, and economic emancipation.[14] Discourses of empowerment among these women also differ from white Western variants of feminism where men are "expunged from feminist spaces and dubbed the enemies."[15]

> The reason for this nonadherence is that most of us do not have jobs because as in our current condition, most of us do not have husbands so our wellbeing is a struggle. We are struggling a lot. It is not easy for us so if the government can employ us, even if it is just small cleaner [janitorial] job in the hospital or local council for us to be able to assist ourselves so we can live our lives progressively. Just as the government has provided free drugs for us, we will also need employment.—[Translated] HIV-seropositive woman

Economic empowerment is also perceived to help confront the real consequences of HIV status disclosure when women fear that they may lose their financial support due to abandonment from divorce or separation. Economic empowerment is thus perceived to enable access to treatment even in the concealment of seropositivity. In cases of nondisclosure of seropositivity, this type of empowerment offers women some level of financial power such that women are capable of initiating treatment and care independent of their partners' knowledge. Economic empowerment also has to be sustainable; hence, the specific reference to government job-type of employment, because, locally, these jobs are longer in tenure and secure, and also come with retirement benefits. This is in contrast to conventional forms of economic empowerment in mainstream development that is practiced through cash transfers and material gifts for income-generating purposes,[16] based on the erroneous supposition that all women possess entrepreneurial experience and skills, thus, undermining long-term economic sustainability when women do not meet up with the business of maintaining income flows.

> If as women, men empower us or we are empowered by ourselves that will be good. Say for example, if I am in my business place, my husband will not know where I go and even the times when I go to access my drugs and also because I am working and bringing my own money. So in this case, I won't have any problem and I will be taking my drugs freely. Even then, I can tell him anything I want and even lie to him that these drugs I am taking are immune balanced diet drugs that I bought [and not ARVs]. I will even be swallowing the drugs in his presence but he can't just ask questions to know the exact nature of the drugs because I purchased them with my money. But just because I am not working now and I am a full housewife, my husband will want to dig to the bottom [question me in-depth] to know the exact nature of the drugs I am swallowing.—[Translated] HIV-seropositive woman

The preceding statement envisions what economic empowerment looks like for women within the context of marriage. Although women's economic autonomy may not fully procure social freedom and the assertion of their rights within marital relationships, it does provide some power and leverage to negotiate gender relations. In this case, it helps women to challenge financial control when it becomes a barrier to access and adherence to ARV treatment. The above quote also asks and engages the obvious, whether economic empowerment may negate HIV status disclosure or enable it. In the current context however, nondisclosure reinforces women's need for economic empowerment and illuminates some of the ways women might deploy their economic power to navigate the treatment terrain especially when their spouses or partners are unaware of their seropositivity.

> The reason why these challenges [to treatment] that we have is very serious is that this thing [HIV/AIDS] can happen to anybody but mostly for us who are poor. The majority of us that are infected are very poor because if a woman has no husband, you know something is wrong [there will be a financial problem], except in situations where a woman has gone to school [educated] and that

> she got an education and was a well-paid worker before the husband dies. So because she earns a salary, she can meet up with the challenges but for us local women like us, it is very difficult for us to meet up [with our needs].—HIV-seropositive woman

Ability to afford housing, transportation, adequate nutrition, and supplementary ARV drugs, as well as childcare, constituted some of the basic needs of HIV-seropositive women that empowerment through employment would help to cater to. Still, the quote above reestablishes the notion that women connect their primary source of economic empowerment to intimate connections with men, especially when women themselves lack education and well-paid, sustainable employment opportunities. It also shows that empowerment for most women is deeply tied to marriage through economic dependence on their husbands, as they cannot as single women realize economic independence without the empowerment that education and sustainable living wage work with benefits can provide them. These doors are closed for poor women, especially those living with HIV. The women, thus, appealed to the Nigerian state and/or NGOs to provide them with dignified work and benefits.

Economic empowerment, although improves women's agency in enabling sustained ARV access, narratives throughout this book indicate that it is not absolute in eliminating all barriers to access and adherence because treatment barriers have been constructed beyond financial constraints even though feminized poverty is a crucial factor. Yet these discourses of empowerment further establish the claim that the concept of empowerment is multidimensional. In addition to illuminating the diverse ways that the concept of empowerment can be referenced and practiced by particular populations, these conceptions also illuminate fundamental policy implications.

Local discourses of needs and empowerment, although characterized by harmful cultural memes that foreground female subservience and patriarchal norms, do expose women's need for social security. Any form of empowerment for women in this context must thus aim to foster their sense of social security within intimate partner and household relations; otherwise, such empowerment programs risk repudiation. It is important to illuminate this because, in this context, most women (and men) identify and believe in female subordination, albeit not intentionally framed as such, but the knowledge that women are subject to the authority of men, thereby subordinate to them in decision-making, is organic to indigenous knowledges and ways of being.

In the Nigerian context, there is also a need to recognize that female empowerment can be undermined by patriarchal power given women's required submission to male authority and the general notion that men have the power to position women either in a state of empowerment or disempowerment. Women's constructions of male superiority foreground their notion of self, how they construct their identities and gender roles, and what their notions of masculinity are in relation to themselves. It is, as have been argued, a function of a dimension of power where the actors lack a consciousness of power hierarchies, of domination and subordination because of deeply entrenched inequalities that are rarely perceived as abnormal, either because both groups are unconscious of their dominate or subordinate positions or because these behaviors are structurally patterned and perceived as organic, thereby, eliminating conflicts.[17] The notion of choices or alternative ways of doing is thus elided as existing norms tend to conceal such possibilities and also because the ability to fulfill the alternative is not only shaped by the availability of resources but also shaped by the perception or knowledge of available choices and resources. This dimension of power is crucial to this analysis and elucidates the importance of a relational model of empowerment that includes both men and women, as well as the idea of empowerment as self-liberation.

Currently, male involvement in HIV/AIDS interventions in Nigeria is weakly referenced in the national strategic action plans. Qualitative evidence from this research shows a perception of gender equity strategies among policy stakeholders as commonly equated with women-focused programs that prioritize women over men. The evidence strengthens the usual arguments for male involvement in women's empowerment programs, whether material or otherwise. By this, men are oriented and enabled to form meaningful partnerships with their spouses and partners in engendering the success of such programs without feelings of marginalization. Yet, in spite of the proven significance of this strategy in reworking gendered inequalities and power,[18] male involvement in Nigerian HIV/AIDS interventions does not seem to have gained much traction. For the most part, it is documented as a strategy in gender policy documents, in particular, Prevention of Mother to Child Transmission (PMTCT) programs but less across other aspects of HIV/AIDS interventions such as treatment. There is ambivalence in the way this strategy is sometimes articulated as important yet peripheral and mostly ignored in program design and implementation because of the ways that policy actors construct empowerment programs in women-specific terms.[19]

Empowerment as self-liberation comes through the elevation of an individual's consciousness and of others through the power of information and knowledge—for men and women—to (re)think and rework unhealthy gender norms such that transformation begins from the mind. Empowerment of the mind represents an ideological shift in gender mapping and orientation for both men and women. Otherwise, gender-specific empowerment programs will at best provide a temporary safety net or solution for women without long-term traction as patriarchal structures remain stable. Empowerment must thus, begin by targeting women's minds (and men) and thought processes to elicit awareness and recognition of more subtle and immanent forms of inequalities, as well as oppressive male behavior, that have mutated overtime to become the norm. It also involves raising women's self-awareness to the recognition of real possibilities of securing social and economic securities outside of traditional sources and spaces, like marriage.

FEMINISM IN NIGERIA

Despite its steeped patriarchal nature, Nigeria has a long history of feminism or what may be referred to in precolonial and colonial times as women activists groups. Informal in structure and not aptly referenced as feminist movements, these groups lobbied and agitated for the rights of women through collective action.[20] Like in many parts of Africa, for example, Ghana and Kenya, there was some semblance of patriarchy in the way that the Nigerian society was organized in the precolonial era. Notwithstanding, the idea of a core patriarchal system became firmly established through the practices of colonial administrators who delegitimized the centrality of women and their contributions to public life in the domains of agriculture, economic production, and political participation.[21]

In South Africa, colonialism not only ushered in modernist political ideologies of liberalism but also instituted a system of indirect rule where power was devolved at the level of male traditional chiefs. Colonialism brought some vestiges of liberalism, but the strategy of indirect rule deployed by the minority male white settlers to keep Africans subjugated, created a level of traditional governance that devolved power to men and shifted meanings of gender rights (and equality) across all spheres of life.[22] Traditional governance structures modeled after white patriarchal dominance with respect to male-led leadership became significant in upholding gendered hierarchies.[23]

Women's movements in the colonial era were thus organized as anti-colonial struggles and in direct resistance to patriarchal authority and colonial interventions that centralized men in the public domain to the detriment of women.[24] The 1929 Aba Women's riot by Igbo female traders in protest against high British taxation is a notable example of organized women's movement and female activism in Nigeria. This trend of established patriarchy and counter-resistance progressed into postcolonial Nigeria with a considerable number of social movements that now intentionally identify and affiliate their interests with women.[25]

The National Council for Women's Societies (NCWS), founded in 1958, is the oldest and largest organized national women's movement in Nigeria but largely criticized for its use of nonconfrontational strategies in resistance to patriarchal oppression.[26] What may be regarded as corporate feminist activism, a politically organized movement and formal constitution of women's social action using legal tools and institutionalized approaches, was formally established in 1983 through the Women in Nigeria (WIN) organization. WIN became the pioneer organization that clearly identified with the feminist label, paving the way for newer organizations like the NFF.[27] The NFF, an outcome of the pan-African Feminist Forum (AFF) that was held in Accra, Ghana, was launched as a core *feminist* movement in 2008, becoming a chapter of the AFF in Nigeria. The NFF is bound by the regional ideologies, principles, and values of the AFF, which are primarily the rights of women and their total emancipation from exploitative and oppressive patriarchal structures.[28]

Although most of the issues the NFF advocates for are local and continental to Nigeria and the African state, respectively, the group also pays a strong commitment to global Western feminist ideals through its charter which espouses the rights to abortion, individual sexual identities and orientation, which for many indigenous feminists are not only less fundamental to the African feminist agenda but also associated with foreign values.[29] African feminist discourses centralize a human rights strategy to promote women's social, political, religious, cultural, legal, and economic rights yet embody class, cultural, and religious interests.[30] African feminism is also essentially natal and heterosexual—a departure from Western feminist engagement with abortion rights and lesbian politics.[31]

In a published journal article by the NFF and one that lays the foundation for this analysis, as it appears to be the only official and publicly available publication from this organization, the NFF explicitly identifies and engages with the subject of feminism in Nigeria, Africa, and the globe. In this article, the NFF attempts to establish itself at the forefront of feminism in Nigeria and positions itself as a core leader in this movement.[32] The NFF asserts that until its launch, WIN was the foremost feminist movement but has now been effectively replaced by the NFF.[33] Although the NFF highlights its shared commonality with WIN in that they are both formally constituted and organized *feminist* movements, it also draws multiple contrasts. To this end, the NFF asserts its clearly well-defined mission and objectives as "larger and more coherent than WIN," and having moved beyond the historical stage of isolated national movements to become part of the continental (pan-African) and global feminist movements.[34] Most importantly, the NFF critiques WIN's open membership policy to individuals with divergent feminist views. In contrast, the NFF has specific guidelines and criteria that define those who can seek membership, foremost of which is to embrace the NFF's feminist ideologies.[35]

The NFF is, thus, a mix of both African and Western feminist ideals not because of its connections to the AFF but because it shares the goals of the broader African feminist struggle or movement, while at the same time, it also embraces third-wave feminist philosophies. The NFF also constructs women's marginal contexts as not been limited to their immediate geographies, but also of invisible flows from global structures and processes that remarginalize women, and which must be accounted for in local feminist struggles—a perspective that is consistent with this book's definition of context.

Also visible in the NFF's publication is a deliberate attempt to use language as a social and political tool to establish its distinct feminist identity and agenda. In their charter, their self-proclaimed identity as "staunch feminists" and assertion of the rights to use the term *feminist*, as African women, can be likened to making a strong social and political statement that resists traditional views associated with the word, "feminism" in Nigeria, as well as a direct repudiation of male power.[36] It conveys the *it is not business as usual* message, because in some feminist circles and notably the NFF's critique of the NCWS, which I discuss later in this section, gender cooperation or any form of perceived diplomacy with men is perceived as pandering to the ideals of patriarchy and, thus, reinforcing male supremacy.

Further analysis of the publication shows that the NFF deploys language and texts politically to label and craft its ideological mission, as well as in their stated struggle "to dismantle patriarchy," in their quest for women's emancipation and empowerment. The NFF's advancement of radical and confrontational feminism, especially through their use of language, also shows the organization's efforts to not only carve a distinct niche in the local feminist scene but also distance itself from what has become the mainstream feminist trend in Nigeria. Although, as I previously argued, there is no absolute body of knowledge that prescribes or defines what Nigerian feminism is. Existing trends across women's movements and schools of thought (many do not explicitly identify as feminist) show essential features of the broader indigenous feminist movement in Nigeria to be mostly nonconfrontational with men and an overall engagement with diplomacy and negotiation. This is not so much a critique of the NFF but a deconstruction of its ideologies and rhetoric and, if they are a legitimate representation of the larger sociocultural configuration of the country considering the level of representation this body seeks, to be the face of the feminist movement in Nigeria.

For example, patriarchy, as defined by the NFF, is a system "of male authority which legitimizes the oppression of women through political, social, economic, legal, cultural, religious and military institutions. . . [and] our ideological task as feminists is to understand this system and our political task is to *end* it. Our focus is *fighting* against patriarchy as a system rather than fighting individual men or women. . . . With this Charter, we reaffirm our commitment to *dismantling* patriarchy in all its manifestations in Africa [emphasis mine]."[37] Because patriarchy is symbolic with male control, although the NFF may frame their mission as not *fighting individual men* but the oppressive practices permeated through its structures, the use of confrontational language may obscure this objective and meet with resistance from men and also women who oppose the use of confrontational politics in feminist activism. Any form of social activism that addresses the oppressive practices of patriarchy is laudable and should be embraced. Nevertheless, the NFF's combative approach does bring up a fundamental issue on effective feminist strategies within patriarchal frameworks and also the implication of radical feminism, especially for women at the grassroots who are still very much trapped in the quagmire of social, ideological, and economic oppression.

Although the NFF's values, which include the respect, defense, and protection of the rights of women, key into fundamental feminist goals, its radical take on feminism or women's empowerment is arguably a far lesser representation of the incredibly diverse groups of women in Nigeria, for example, the voices of HIV-seropositive women understudied. This is one of the reasons why feminism in Nigeria has come to be perceived as the purview of a crop of educated and privileged women because sometimes, its discourse and practices are exclusionary of other gendered worldviews and, therefore, inimical to the shared goal of emancipation for all women.

Any discourse on women's empowerment that appears to repudiate male authority or leadership may not be directly beneficial to women at the grassroots, especially peasant women, who constitute a majority of the women population that are yet to fully develop their sense of self or articulate their autonomy from male power. This is not to say that poor women do not try to resist micro-level male dominations and inequalities especially within household relations but this is mostly performed using less contentious approaches as we see in the narratives of HIV-seropositive women.[38] Anti-feminist discourses are thus rife among the local population as a female community health worker at the Erhoike health center opined.

> It is [gender] still an issue, it is still an issue because the issue of gender, the men still want to tell you that they are the big shots [so] whatever they tell you as the wife, you will take. . . . The public enlightenment [on gender equality], most men frown at it [saying] that these are foreign culture [and that] they should not bring the foreign culture into Nigeria. If you as a woman, you are buying [into] the gender equality [agenda], your husband will start telling you that you are following this foreign culture [and] you cannot exhibit it in my house [because] I am an African man [and] you are supposed to be an African woman. We have our culture; we have to follow our culture. So for the equity to really stand, I think it is common with the educated ones who have really gone out [exposed to

western cultures] and they have really bought that idea but I think it's something that we [locals] are still battling in this environment to buy [into] that idea but I don't really know how soon we will buy it.—Community health worker

This excerpt makes a reference to the distinct ways that individuals at the grassroots and the more elite perceive gender equality and female empowerment, with education, social and class privileges seen as fundamental to this difference. For the former group, it is the notion of foreignness and cultural imperialism, and, thus, feminism meets with rejection. The assertion of education, social and class privileges as key exposures to identifying with and embracing the values of feminism is also backed by evidence in the scholarship. For example, many African and Nigerian female literary scholars who form part of this elite group are now coming to terms with the concept of feminism, partly due to the redefinition of feminism on African terms and values.[39]

While the privileged locations of this group of women literary writers may have played a role in their exposure and acceptance of feminism, their models of feminism—womanism, motherism, stiwanism, nego-feminism, and snail-sense feminism—are nevertheless inherently conservative, with their models described as reformist rather than transformative.[40] Their ideologies have also been critiqued for taking a conciliatory and apologetic stance toward female liberation. This is especially so, given their orientation toward the preservation of African traditions and culture, and sometimes religious values, as opposed to the NFF's more radical approach to feminism which loosely identifies with the fundamentals of religion and culture.[41]

It is important to point out here that although the discourses of empowerment among HIV-seropositive women do not fall neatly into any of the strands of feminism aforementioned, we can, nevertheless, draw key connections—for example, the recognition and accommodation of men in the discourse and practice of female empowerment, as well as the centralization of the culture and values of marriage, family, and motherhood. In this sense, the class and social lines between HIV-seropositive women and the proponents of these indigenous feminist models who are part of the elite are blurred, as these entrenched cultural values and traditions appear to take precedence.

The lines become visible, however, when we juxtapose the narrowly conceived form of empowerment by HIV-seropositive women, which is primarily economic, to the broader conceptions of empowerment and female liberation by elite women. It is at this point that the lack of education and other forms of exposure appear to influence how most of the HIV-seropositive women conceived empowerment. This is in addition to their experiences of household and intimate relationships where the women perceived their lack of or poor economic power as a primary factor that adversely regulates their everyday lives and social realities.

On the other hand, the NFF's discourse parallels these popular indigenous feminist models as aforementioned, in the range of issues embraced, especially those that conflict with the fundamental values of the mainstream culture and religion in Nigeria, like abortion and gay rights, and which can be attributed to their affiliation with the global feminist movement. For example, in critiquing what it cites as a deficiency of traditional women's movements like the NCWS, the NFF states:[42]

> This movement [NCWS] is "at home" with the protection of our culture and tradition as well as with the supremacy of men. It will not rock the boat. It essentially accepts what the tradition has been and what religion sanctions.

Nigeria as a male-dominated society with vital aspects of its culture deeply embedded in patriarchal structures is a fact that has been stressed throughout this book. Still, it is reductionist to sum the local culture and tradition in essentialist patriarchal terms, thereby, obscuring other valued aspects of culture. While patriarchy is predominantly intertwined with the mainstream culture, values like family, respect, sharing, and communality, among others, are independent of patriarchy. A radical approach to contest local ideologies of tradition may end up reproducing the structures that feminist movements aim to destabilize because what is gained becomes resistance to change not just by men but also by women—the subjects or groups purportedly represented and advocated for. As women in patriarchal contexts, whose histories and daily lives are marked with the concrete experiences of female subordination, it is easy to be swept in the whirlwind of extreme emotions that the struggle for emancipation may provoke. But combative and exclusionary discourses also produce the risk of losing the critical edge of this struggle and consequently undermining the important goal of transforming the unequal relations between women and men.

The current discourse also illuminates issues on representation, needs, interests, and inclusion, for example, which categories of women are included or excluded from the broader indigenous feminist movement as the agenda of particular feminist movements such as the NFF becomes popular, not because of its vast ideological representation but for its voice. Indigenous feminists, thus, fall into the trap of reproducing differences among women along education, social, and class lines, because their discourses are sometimes exclusive of the voices of peasant women, like this group of HIV-seropositive women. These women simply desire to be empowered with the material ability to make independent choices but without jeopardizing the security of their intimate relationships which may occur through an aggressive stance against male authority.

The discourses of both elite and peasant women point toward the common goal of empowerment for the Nigerian woman but with conceptual and practical differences on the path to actualization. As have been argued, feminism cannot be defined in hegemonic or imperialistic terms without it been contradictory to the very ideals that it espouses, which is liberation, especially if women being represented feel that particular praxes of feminism are antithetical to their own beliefs and values. While the fluidity of gender and the diverse ways it is experienced by culture, geography, and other markers of difference makes it challenging or even impossible to identify a form of feminism that is homogenous to all women, perhaps, this inherent diversity is what makes the feminist movement unique. Still, feminist researchers and activists must find practical ways to forge an inclusive path to the freedom and empowerment of women, regardless of their social, class, religious, and cultural locations.

A truly representational feminism does not preclude difference but it does not define and impose its conception of liberation based on the subjectivities, interests, and social consciousness of specific groups. Rather, it centralizes its focus on the liberation and empowerment of the mind in ways that enable individual self-awareness and identities, as well as the consciousness and ability of women to make choices in an environment that is free from negative influence, control, and manipulation.

Like feminism, the concept of women's empowerment is steeped in complicity with connections to geography, culture, and social locations. This complexity has produced varied discourses of empowerment in the present context. Among the cohort of HIV-seropositive women investigated, economic sustainability and social security are the key elements they associate with empowerment. That is, empowerment must be sustainable in the long term and also ensure their socioeconomic security within the household. Although the form of empowerment that is pushed for by these women, such that they are economically empowered but ignore socially oppressive conditions, is inimical to transformative gender development, it is the voices of such women that we need to listen to. Not because their partial and distorted views of gender and social relations should be considered normative or authoritative knowledge but silencing these voices through exclusionary ideologies and combative feminist discourses will not produce the transformation that is especially needed at the grassroots.

Feminists' calls to alter traditional and mainstream epistemologies for the production of locally situated knowledge reinforce this position. For example, Nalia Kabeer posits that locally situated knowledge is that "which emerges out of experience rather than theory, although it may inform and improve theory."[43] It is, thus, derived from the direct experiences of subjects shaped by the unique processes and characteristics of places. It is from the vantage perspectives of marginalized subjects and groups that the intricacies of subordination and oppression can be fully grasped and better utilized to reconstruct more equitable structures so that development policies and practices can closely mirror the "real order of things."[44]

Empowerment initiatives must thus take into cognizance the multiple subjectivities of target populations and other forms of hierarchy and difference through an inclusive gender approach, in order to establish a more egalitarian society where women like men have equal opportunities and access to resources, and are able to attain any level of citizenship and individuality so desired. I argue, nevertheless, that it is more effective to work through the cracks and fault lines of a society to transform or modify its culture because to aim to tumultuously usurp the existing *status quo* as radical feminists claim, is not only unrealistic but also self-defeating.

I am not advocating a double speak on the issue. I do not in the least even propose a movement that is complacent to patriarchy or fails to critique existing power structures. Rather, resistance to patriarchal structures that undermine women's autonomy should be a progressive and systematic process, using tools and strategies that are far more reaching and inclusive to prevent undue resistance to the agenda of social transformation by the actual agents of change.

NOTES

1. Ama Ata Aidoo A, "Unwelcome Pals and Decorative Slaves - or Glimpses of Women as Writers and Characters in Contemporary African Literature," in *Literature and Society: Selected Essays on African Literature*, ed. Ernest Emeyonu (Oguta: Zim Pan African Publishers, 1989), 34.

2. Nalia Kabeer, *Reversed Realities: Gender, Hierarchies in Development Thought* (London: Verso, 1994), 33. Also see dependency theory arguments by Don D. Marshall, "The New World Group of Dependency Scholars," in *The Companion to Development Studies*, eds. Vandana Desai and Robert B. Potter (London: Routledge, 2014), 189; and James D. Sidaway, "Post-Development," in *The Companion to Development Studies*, eds. Vandana Desai and Robert B. Potter (London: Routledge, 2014), 228.

3. See Nalia Kabeer, "Gender Equality and Women's Empowerment: A Critical Analysis of the Third Millennium Development Goal," *Gender and Development* 13, no. 1 (March 2005): 14, https://doi.org/10.1080/13552070512331332273.

4. Susan Arndt, "African Gender Trouble and African Womanism: An Interview with Chikwenye Ogunyemi and Wanjira Muthoni," *Signs* 25, no. 3 (Spring 2000): 710; Mary Kolawole, "Transcending Incongruities: Rethinking Feminism and the Dynamics of Identity in Africa," *Agenda: Empowering Women for Gender Equity* 17, no. 54 (2002): 92, https://doi.org/10.1080/10130950.2002.9676183.

5. See Susan Arndt, "Perspectives on African Feminism: Defining and Classifying African Feminist Literatures," *Agenda: Empowering Women for Gender Equity* 17, no. 54 (2002): 31–32, https://doi.org/10.1080/10130950.2002.9676176.

6. See Naomi Nkealah, "(West) African Feminisms and Their Challenges," *Journal of Literary Studies* 32, no. 2 (2016): 62, https://doi/org/10.1080/02564718.2016.1198156.

7. See Arndt, "Perspectives on African Feminism," 31; Arndt, "African Gender Trouble and African Womanism," 710.

8. Nkealah, "(West) African Feminisms and Their Challenges," 62, 64.

9. Ibid., 63–68. For further notes on each of these variants, see Catherine Obianuju Acholonu, *Motherism: The Afrocentric Alternative to Feminism* (Owerri: Afa Publications, 1995); Mary Modupe Kolawole, *Womanism and African Consciousness* (Eritrea: Africa World Press, 1997); Molara Ogundipe-Leslie, *Re-Creating Ourselves: African Women and Critical Transformations* (Trenton, NJ: Africa World Press, 1994); see Obioma Nnaemeka, "Nego-Feminism: Theorizing, Practicing and Pruning Africa's Way," *Signs: Journal of Women in Culture and Society* 29, no. 2 (2003) and Akachi Ezeigbo, *Snail-Sense Feminism: Building on an Indigenous Model* (Lagos: University of Lagos, 2012).

10. Nkealah, "(West) African Feminisms and Their Challenges," 63–65. Also see Kolawole, "Transcending Incongruities," 95–96.

11. Kabeer, *Reversed Realities*, 13.

12. Ibid., 7.

13. Elisabeth Porter, "Rethinking Women's Empowerment," *Journal of Peacebuilding and Development* 8, no. 1 (July 2013): 3, https://doi.org/10.1080/15423166.2013.785657.

14. See Kolawole, "Transcending Incongruities," 95; Arndt, "Perspectives on African Feminism," 32.

15. Nkealah, "(West) African Feminisms and Their Challenges," 62.

16. Porter, "Rethinking Women's Empowerment," 4.

17. For the purpose of this analysis, the three dimensions of power identified here are combined from Kabeer, *Reversed Realities*, 226–227 and Lukes Steven's three dimensions of power, in Jacques Charmes and Saskia Wieringa, "Measuring Women's Empowerment: An Assessment of the Gender-Related Development Index and the Gender Empowerment Measurement," *Journal of Human Development* 4, no. 3 (November 2003): 422, https://doi.org/10.1080/1464988032000125773.

18. For example, see Wessel van den Berg et al., "Improving Men's Participation in Preventing Mother-to-Child Transmission of HIV as a Maternal, Neonatal, and Child Health Priority in South Africa," *PloS Medicine* 12, no. 4 (April 2015), https://doi.org/10.1371/journal.pmed.1001811.

19. See Sarah J. Hawkes and Kent Buse, "Gender and Global Health: Evidence, Policy and Inconvenient Truths," *The Lancet* 381 (2013): 1785.

20. Abdul et al., *Analysis of the History, Organizations and Challenges of Feminism in Nigeria* (Spanish Agency for International Development Cooperation, 2012), 5.

21. Nkolika Ijeoma Aniekwu, "Converging Constructions: A Perspective on Sexuality and Feminism in Post-Colonial Africa," *African Sociological Review* 10, no. 1 (2006): 148.

22. Mark Hunter, *Love in the Time of AIDS: Inequality, Gender and Rights in South Africa* (Bloomington: Indiana University Press, 2010), 8.

23. Ibid., 8.

24. Abdul et al., *Analysis of the History of Feminism in Nigeria*, 5.

25. Simidele Dosekun, "Defending Feminism in Africa," *Postamble* 3, no. 1 (2007): 44; Abdul et al., *Analysis of the History of Feminism in Nigeria*, 290.

26. Ayesha, M. Imam, "The Dynamics of WINning: An Analysis of Women in Nigeria (WIN)," in *Feminist Genealogies, Colonial Legacies, Democratic Futures*, eds. M. Jacqui Alexander and Chandra Talpade Mohanty (New York: Routledge, 1997), 296.

27. Abdul et al., *Analysis of the History of Feminism in Nigeria*, 7. Also see Bene E. Madunagu, "The Nigerian Feminist Movement: Lessons from Women in Nigeria, WIN," *Review of African Political Economy* 35, no. 118 (2008): 666.

28. Ibid., 668–670.

29. See Arndt, "African Gender Trouble and African Womanism," 712; Aniekwu, "Converging Constructions," 143–144.

30. Ibid., 143.

31. Ibid.

32. Madunagu, "The Nigerian Feminist Movement," 672.

33. Ibid., 668.

34. Ibid.

35. Ibid., 667–668.

36. The word "feminism" in many African countries, including Nigeria, is foreign not because it is unheard of but for its perceived association with imperialistic Western values that undermine African (or Nigerian) values and culture.

37. Madunagu, "The Nigerian Feminist Movement," 670; emphasis in the quote is the author's.

38. Also see Aniekwu, "Converging Constructions."

39. Kolawole, "Transcending Incongruities," 93.

40. See Arndt, "Perspectives on African Feminism," 33.

41. See Madunagu, "The Nigerian Feminist Movement," 666, 671.

42. Ibid., 666.

43. Kabeer, *Reversed Realities*, 82.

44. Ibid., 81.

Chapter 7

Biomedicalization of Treatment Interventions and HIV/AIDS Support Networks

The meeting place of the Courage HIV/AIDS support group, although located in a remote corner on the grounds of the Erhoike health center, is central to the lives of the cohort of twenty-two HIV-seropositive women who sat down together with me, twice and with multiple follow-up interviews within a four-month period, to share their most intimate experiences of living with HIV in the Niger Delta region. This space exemplifies many things but more than anything, it embodies survival and hope for the many HIV-infected individuals, mostly women, who have turned to it for support.

In one of the monthly support group meetings of about twenty people in attendance, of which only two were males, I had a deeply emotional experience sitting and observing a group of people whose main connection was in the experience of a debilitating virus, yet forging a common goal of survival, hope, and fortitude. My academic training and prior professional experience had not adequately prepared me with the skills to maneuver my emotions

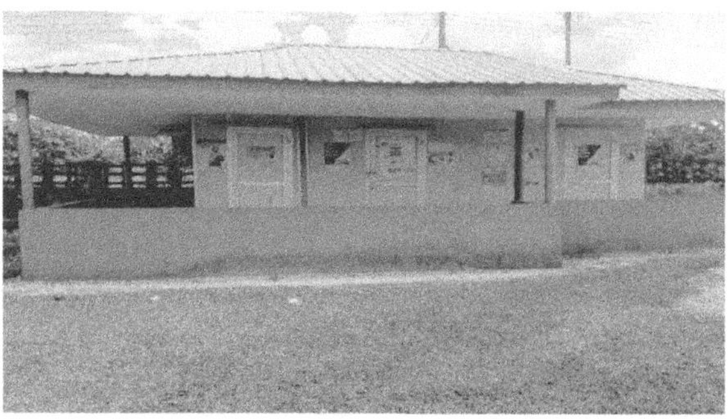

Figure 7.1. The Courage HIV/AIDS support group.
Source: Author, personal photography.

and negotiate this profound moment as I observed the strong bond, and the psychosocial and emotional support that members rendered each other. As a researcher, it was a moment of deep reflexivity and one that also brought in the self-consciousness of an outsider privileged to share in the feelings and experiences of women who did not intentionally choose their biological predicament. And as an insider, being indigenous, it was easy to make connections with these women who embodied the same place history and marginalizing structures that have come to form an intrinsic part of our identities.

The two female leaders of the group, also HIV-seropositive, gave a health talk that was more of a pep talk. Thereafter, members were requested to provide feedback on their health and welfare. Some members complained of the side effects of the drugs and the drudgery of taking ARV drugs for life. Others raised issues of HIV-status disclosure, financial hardships, and the ways that these undermined both their access and adherence to treatment. The leaders followed up these complaints with further counseling and stressed the need for members to adhere to their treatment, in spite of the challenges, in order to achieve and maintain a strong biological immunity to the virus.

At the meeting, members also shared personal stories that depicted strategies and skills that they deployed daily to navigate their seropositivity. These stories were motivational and appeared to aim at personally inspiring members to maintain a healthy and positive attitude. From members' responses, these stories inspired feelings of hope, resilience, and strength through memes that centralized God, faith, and miracles. Some members expressed belief in a higher supernatural power that would eventually make possible a cure for HIV/AIDS and relied on this faith to cope daily with their predicament. It was apparent that members of the support group depended on each other for psychosocial support.

For many women accessing treatment at the Erhoike health center, this is what the Courage HIV/AIDS support group embodies—an alternative resource center that is both a caring space and a site for the accumulation of psychosocial and material capital. The kind of resources provided by HIV/AIDS support groups, in general, is the most commonly cited reason that these groups have become a popular and major coping pathway for seropositive individuals, especially in spaces where biomedical interventions fail to bridge the social gaps in treatment.[1]

Previous chapters uncovered the ways that gendered barriers and structural constraints help us understand why HIV-seropositive women shun free treatment even at their own peril. This chapter explores a major mechanism—HIV/AIDS support groups—by which HIV-seropositive women negotiate these barriers and why this space is of utmost importance to this population. The analysis is developed around the Courage HIV/AIDS support group (domiciled at the Erhoike health center), which is also part of a larger support system and network of HIV-infected individuals nationwide. HIV-seropositive women's testimonies reveal the centrality of therapeutic care and socioeconomic aid provided through the support group as significant points of entry into their coping with HIV.

HIV/AIDS support groups are an unofficial arm of the HIV treatment landscape, unofficial because the Network of People Living with HIV/AIDS in Nigeria (NEPWHAN)—the central coordinating body of all HIV/AIDS support groups—although officially recognized and established as a non-state actor is not incorporated as a formal body or arm of the country's HIV/AIDS intervention system.[2] This network which was formally established in 1998, aims to provide support services to members and protect the rights of people living with HIV/AIDS in Nigeria.[3] It comprises smaller HIV/AIDS support groups at the grassroots which like the Courage HIV/AIDS support group, originally emerged to provide follow-up services to patients, in order to ensure strict compliance with treatment protocols. With time however, the operative scope of these support groups especially at the national level has been reconfigured by the nature of members' needs to provide advocacy and collaboration with HIV/AIDS policy-related interventions, especially with the current limits of biomedical interventions.

From women's perspectives, HIV/AIDS support groups are fast becoming critical circuits of care, and social and material capital within the mainstream HIV/AIDS intervention landscape. From a structural perspective, the push-pull factors to the Courage HIV/AIDS support group not only legitimize the unmet needs of women living with HIV but reveal limited access to such resources in the mainstream society. In addition, the internal dynamics of the support group are also shaped by gender and class-based inequalities.

I use the Courage HIV/AIDS support group to draw attention to the ways that HIV/AIDS support networks are being transformed and reconstituted by prevailing class, social and gender inequalities, as well as their mutually constitutive relationship with members and the broader treatment landscape. The chapter also elucidates the different ways that the Courage HIV/AIDS support group is positively transforming the lives of *unhealthy* subjects as its services act as the missing but important nexus between the gendered bodies of HIV subjects and the biomedicalization of treatment interventions. Although poorly funded, the reported positive impacts of the HIV/AIDS support group intensify the need to strengthen its capacity and service delivery mechanisms, with a recommendation to formally institutionalize its broader network as an official arm of the HIV/AIDS intervention system, as well as expand its coverage at the grassroots.

HIV women's unmet social and material needs as they undermine treatment, also draw attention to the weaknesses of interventions articulated through women's perceptions and assessments of current HIV/AIDS programs. Limited psychosocial and economic resources provided by HIV/AIDS interventions as well as practices that exclude recipients from being mainstreamed into the policy and planning processes formed important critiques. HIV-seropositive women blamed their unaddressed needs on the disconnect between their needs and the priorities of donor agencies, and argued for a more inclusive and active involvement in intervention planning, as well as direct access to policy stakeholders.

Based on the evidence, this chapter also makes the claim that interventions are often out of sync with HIV subjects with three notable kinds of disconnect: structural, ideological, and substantive. Current interventions do not actually mirror the structural realities of marginalized women. Similarly, women's social and material conceptualizations of needs and access at the grassroots are ideologically unaligned with dominant biomedical regimes. Consequently, the substantive resources that accrue from biomedical interventions become less efficient in addressing women's psychosocial and material needs to maintain treatment access and adherence.

HIV/AIDS SUPPORT GROUPS AS EMERGING THERAPEUTIC ENCLAVES

Women's experiential accounts of treatment establish that the convolution of barriers that challenge their access and adherence are best understood within a structural and non-biomedical framework. It is pertinent to state that the propositions made in this book are not against the use of biomedical solutions to address public health problems; in lieu, the argument is that biomedical solutions should not be constructed as universal and hegemonic, especially in contexts where such solutions do not suffice.

Analyzing and interpreting individual treatment risks within a structural framework does not preclude the notion of individual strategies to negotiate and cope with structural constraints. Along this line, women's testimonies demonstrate a quest and acquisition of coping and survival strategies, albeit within a narrow range of opportunities. An important survival mechanism for HIV-seropositive individuals, as previously mentioned, is finding safe spaces through social groups and networks of people with shared interests and commonality. HIV/AIDS support groups usher infected individuals into a space of belonging. Hence, a critical appraisal of these groups' activities, funding, and organizational structure is pertinent to further advance knowledge on their role and importance to HIV/AIDS interventions, despite their non-state nature.

Although unofficial and with a nonprofit structure, HIV/AIDS support groups are very critical to the Nigerian HIV/AIDS intervention chain because of the kind of support services, both socioeconomic and policy, that they render to the body of infected individuals.[4] But their non-state nature means that there is no mandated funding mechanism for them through traditional funding systems or state machineries. At best, more established HIV/AIDS support groups or networks usually at the national level like NEPWHAN, are able to independently attract funds from donor agencies to help coordinate their activities and assist local support groups registered with them to achieve prevention, comprehensive care, and support for members.[5] In contrast, however, many grassroots HIV/AIDS support groups like the Courage support group are unable to attract such funding except as secondary beneficiaries of networks like NEPWHAN and from donor resources channeled through NGOs.

HIV/AIDS support groups compensate for the overly biomedical paradigm of HIV/AIDS programs by completing the intervention chain through a holistic and comprehensive approach to HIV/AIDS service delivery. While the establishment of support groups in treatment facilities appears to be a general recognition of their importance, this is contradicted by poor funding and the lackluster approach by relevant institutional actors. With depleting funds from existing donor-sponsored NGO programs, the Courage HIV/AIDS support group, for example, is on the verge of extinction because of financial challenges, which will eventually pose consequences for seropositive women whose access and adherence to treatment are contingent on the support they receive from this group. The leaders of this group, also HIV-seropositive women, have, thus, sometimes felt compelled to personally bear the financial cost of supporting their distressed members, providing care that extends beyond their original jurisdiction and mandate. These leaders, although financially inadequate, perform such care because over time they have become personally invested in the lives of the people they support. Given the high performativity of support groups, in general, and the resources they generate for the underserved HIV-seropositive population, it is safe to argue that their exclusion from mainstream funding plans is a huge omission and flaw in the HIV/AIDS intervention framework.

Policy stakeholders and women living with HIV brand HIV/AIDS support groups as the most significant channel for negotiating stigma and drug-related barriers to treatment. A deeper analysis, however, reveals other motivations that are complicit in the deficit of social and material capital from interventions, which also explain why this space has become very pivotal to HIV-seropositive individuals, especially women. For example, significant push factors to the Courage HIV/AIDS support group include dissatisfaction with the nature and delivery of services procured through the Erhoike health center. In this sense, the HIV-seropositive women critiqued the overemphasis on drugs to the detriment of socioeconomic considerations that challenged ARV uptake. Psychosocial services like counseling and therapy were also deemed suboptimal.

HIV-seropositive women described some of the healthcare workers as hostile, unsupportive, and unwelcoming to patients. The general level of mistrust between patients and healthcare workers thus compels the support group leaders to function as liaisons or middlemen to bridge the "us and them" gap that seropositive women referenced, in what Ian Hodgson refers to as the "social distance" between health-challenged subjects and health workers.[6] Through the group's monthly gathering, leaders also work to create a space of acceptance and belonging for patients who feel particularly vulnerable and outcast from their families and mainstream society through the impartation of psychosocial skills and coping strategies. In this way, HIV patients regain their lost self-esteem and sense of self, and are socially normalized and reorientated into society.

> Yes, the women I have seen that do come to access drugs in this hospital, they prefer coming to us [support group leaders], wanting us to attend to them. . . . Like since we started working here, most of them [HIV-seropositive women], when they discover we are here, have been able to gather that courage of feeling at home and being more comfortable with themselves in terms of accessing the drugs and they have been able to move on with their lives. They are happy about it.—HIV-seropositive woman and support group leader

Support group leaders double as biological and socioeconomic risk managers. Besides the medical support they provide, for example, assisting members with their prescriptions and dealing with drug side effects, they also support women with funds for transportation and supplementary treatment drugs like multivitamins that are not free to HIV patients. Financial support is provided to new mothers and members in bereavement. Psychosocially, the group helps women in the self-management of living with HIV, assists members to resolve issues of (non)disclosure, empowers women to fight stigma through health education and awareness, and inspires growth and development of self-confidence as well as find social acceptance within and outside the group. For some women, their marriages and homes have been salvaged through the interventions of the support group as they learned and acquired coping skills and strategies in dealing with their day-to-day struggles. A majority of the women reportedly gained emotional and psychological stability, self-confidence, and a broadened knowledge of the infection and disease through the support group.

> I enjoy the support group because when I just came into this hospital to begin accessing my drugs, I was told that there is a support group that helps people access and adhere to their drugs. I decided that I would like to join. It was when

I joined the meeting that I rebuilt my self-confidence. Before now, even after the doctors and health workers have counseled me, when I got home, I still thought about my situation and sometimes, I thought and asked myself, if this is the way I will continue to take these drugs until my death? But since I began attending the meeting, I started seeing people who are fat because I used to think that it was this sickness that made me to be slim but when I started seeing people who are taking these drugs and yet looking fat and robust, I knew that my slimness was just as a result of my genes. When I started this meeting I said to myself, if these people that are on these medications look like this and they live their lives freely and don't think about this HIV, I can also take these medications consistently, and also attend the meetings.—[Translated] HIV-seropositive woman

Despite these gains, the notion that the support group is an alternative care space to the main treatment facility does not hold true for all HIV-infected persons. Not all HIV-seropositive women or men benefit or access resources from this group. Members' demographics offer some insights into some of the conditions that designate the support group as a safe space and by whom; that is, the category of infected persons most likely to value and engage this space to accumulate psychosocial and economic capital outside the health facility, household, and other spaces. Members' demographics reveal that gender- and class-based identities are strong push-pull factors. At the Erhoike health center, although every HIV patient is expected to be a member of the support group (see Figure 7.2), observations and reports indicate that membership is a homogenous pattern of mostly peasant women, with men and middle-to upper-class educated women relatively absent.

Poverty is a major push factor and motivation for support group participation. The heavy presence of women in the group may be affirmative of prevailing socioeconomic disparities that impact women more than men in this geography. As women's accounts demonstrate, less materially empowered women are more willing to invest time and even obtain small loans from friends and families to attend the monthly meetings as long as the group assured them of financial remuneration. Attendance at the group's monthly meetings had however, visibly thinned out due to depleted funds to the group from

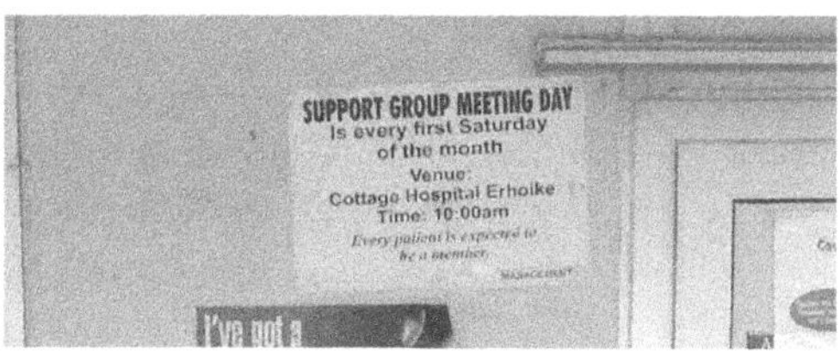
SUPPORT GROUP MEETING DAY
Is every first Saturday
of the month
Venue:
Cottage Hospital Erhoike
Time: 10:00am
I've got a

Figure 7.2 Notice of monthly meeting by the Courage HIV/AIDS support group.
Source: Author, personal photography.

NGOs associated with the health facility. Hence, the treatment facility was no longer able to make funds available to the group for the usual material assistance to members to cover lunch and transportation costs, among other benefits.

> Yes, even yesterday when I called members to tell them that there is a meeting and that they should attend, they were asking me, is there money? They said they did not have transportation and if there is no money, they would not be able to come . . . but if there is money, you will see more than fifty people here but since there is no money, we only have few members in attendance. However, I still do encourage them to come for meetings whether there is money or not.—[Translated] HIV-seropositive woman and support group leader

While the lack of funds constrains attendance to meeting, members are unwilling to attend meetings if they perceive that they may not be reimbursed in amounts greater than their actual cost of transportation. This was the scenario during the recruitment of participants for the focus group discussions. Many of the women had *logically* asked the group's leaders who assisted in the recruitment process if transportation costs would be more than compensated, to ascertain if there was extra cash to be gained. In contrast, the group's leaders appeared to be more altruistic, demonstrated by their decision to continue to offer their services to the group even after their monthly remunerations from the facility ceased. For these leaders, whose financial status can also be compared to the members they serve, their commitment is borne out of a deep sense of purpose, to encourage and enable other women like them to live positively and achieve their full potentials, in spite of their seropositivity. Sometimes this meant taking financial and social responsibility for the welfare of others.

> As an executive [support group leader], it is a voluntary work so I don't expect to gain from what I am doing. I expect to give out the little I have and to see people get well. Those that are living with the virus, I really want to see them happy, at least I really want to see them better and not die like that.—HIV-seropositive woman and support group leader

Altruism is, however, not a value that is shared across all support groups, as one of the leaders in the Courage HIV/AIDS support group mentioned, as she narrated instances where leaders in other support groups have only taken up the role of leadership as a means to earn a livelihood. While incentives to join the group may vary across members and leaders, the support group as an informal financial port especially for women who have few options for a viable livelihood is not in doubt.

Besides the financial incentives, the Courage HIV/AIDS support group also serves as a therapeutic space for members.

> The meetings have really helped me a lot. Even my husband now attends the meetings with me because he knows the meetings help me a lot. I don't worry anymore, I am okay now. I gave birth to a baby and when the baby was HIV-free, it also helped to strengthen my mind a lot and that was when my husband said that this meeting that you are attending that has helped you overcome your moodiness and psychological distress, I also want to attend so that I can learn new things and that is why anytime I come for the meeting, he joins me, we come together.—[Translated] HIV-seropositive woman and support group leader

The support group as a social and therapeutic enclave for mostly women is, however, not unresponsive to structural flows whether in terms of gender, social- and class-based inequalities, or gaps in the current standardized biomedical model of health care which have transformed HIV/AIDS support groups to alternative care sites within the larger healthcare system. The feminized nature of the support group also strengthens the evidence that the challenges to women's access and adherence to treatment are significantly gendered. A paramount reason that explains this is that provisions to women's treatment needs are not always available and accessible to women in the private and public domains of households and mainstream society, as well as health facilities. In fact, existing treatment interventions are such that women access mostly medical services from health facilities but access nonmedical resources from the HIV/AIDS support group.

Perhaps too, the sense of safety that women feel in the Courage HIV/AIDS support group is also a reflection of the visible absence of male power, given that leadership is by women and membership is predominantly female. It is not clear from the available evidence in this study, if having a predominantly male HIV/AIDS support group system with male leadership will change the dynamics and sense of safety that most women have come to associate with this group, in other words, if the prevailing social ethos and gender prejudices will be injected into this space or if members' shared seropositivity will eliminate or even mitigate gender biases. As a result, I theorize with caution that the present *status quo* of this space may represent for HIV-seropositive women some sort of temporary autonomy from patriarchal privilege; hence, the women support group leaders who double as resource managers are able to deploy capital to meet the needs of other women in the group.

The notion that cultural discourses around masculinities and health-seeking behavior are some reasons men may shy away from identification with and active involvement in the support group is also alluded to by the support group leaders. Culturally, negative discourses surround men seeking health care, with such men regarded as weak. The evidence illuminates the role of gender in determining who may or may not access certain kinds of health interventions, in particular, HIV/AIDS support group services.

With mostly poor, uneducated, and rural women seeking care and support from the Courage HIV/AIDS support group, class, social, and gender locations appear to constitute an identity framework that mediates the categories of people who collectively benefit from HIV/AIDS support groups. This is not to propose that women of high socioeconomic class do not offer active membership in support groups particularly in more urban spaces. Perhaps, elite women are able to independently negotiate the social and material challenges of living with HIV without the need to identify with local groups for support, as further conversations with the support group leaders revealed. For elite women, local health groups may not be accorded much importance because they are able to seek and purchase needed benefits through more sophisticated means, for example, professional therapy.

Studies on HIV/AIDS support groups and how they shape the HIV/AIDS community are very scarce, especially in the Nigerian context. Consequently, it is hard to determine the impact of location, whether rural or urban, gender, and other markers of social difference on the structure of support groups in other geographies. What can be argued based on the available evidence is that membership in the Courage HIV/AIDS support group is a deliberate and strategic decision influenced by shared identities, a coalition of common minds, a shared biosocial experience of the infection, as well as real and perceived therapeutic, social, and material benefits.

The emphasis on the support group as the most significant coping outlet by HIV-seropositive women makes it apparent that this space provides a range of services that are beyond the reach of women who turn to it for provision. It is also indicative of the linear nature of HIV treatment interventions to which women offer their perceptions.

PERCEPTIONS OF HIV/AIDS POLICIES AND PROGRAMS

HIV-seropositive women provided a mixed perception of HIV/AIDS interventions. Positive evaluations of HIV/AIDS interventions included the provision of jobs for HIV-seropositive individuals as adherence counselors in the HIV/AIDS support group as well as free ARVs, even though many wished the supplementary drugs were also free.

The most cited weakness of HIV/AIDS interventions is the disjuncture between the nature of intervention resources and the needs of HIV patients. HIV-seropositive women attributed this disconnect to NGOs' priorities. Although a generality of the women voiced their grievances against state

HIV/AIDS institutions, the support group leaders, for instance, expressed their discontent with NGOs. This may be because NGOs are the more visible actors in the geography of HIV/AIDS interventions compared to state actors or agencies. Similarly, NGOs are more accessible to the support group members particularly the group's leaders during monitoring and evaluation of programs, when NGOs visit the health facility. Nevertheless, many of the women perceived this practice as rudimentary and unproductive because NGOs' priorities are donor-oriented and will only respond to women's reported needs when these align with their program requirements.

NGOs were framed as "uncaring" but were generally perceived to be better than state agencies. NGOs were critiqued for having priorities in conflict with patients' needs, with an overemphasis on patients' reports and statistics but less concern about the efficacy of interventions on patients. The women expressed a general distrust of NGOs with claims that NGOs' real motives, although obscured, are less about their welfare. NGOs were argued to *doing the talk* but not fulfilling promises made to patients, and also as exploitative, in that they used patients' statistics to fulfill their own agenda and meet funders' requirements. The women also claimed that both NGOs and state institutions are insensitive to the needs of patients, and blamed state institutions for nonpayment of salaries to HIV/AIDS support group leaders and inadequate training of local health workers to effectively perform their jobs.

Negative perceptions of interventions also included poor representation of patients' needs, and patients' marginalization and exclusion from active involvement in a process that determined their health. Some of the women attributed the disconnect between their needs and interventions to limited access to policy and program stakeholders, and current exclusionary practices that do not enable patients to have direct access to policy stakeholders except through health workers who may not accurately represent patients' interests.

> We don't want them [relevant policy stakeholders and NGOs] to send anybody. We want to talk to them, face to face because the ones they are sending [third party representatives], it is what is on their mind, that is what they are doing, just for their own pocket [financial gain] because I have gone for a seminar like that, it is for the man's own pocket. Even for everything I said [at this seminar], I have not heard anything [feedback]. So we want to talk to them [relevant stakeholders and institutions] one on one.—HIV-seropositive woman and support group leader

HIV-seropositive women described effective policy access in terms of organized forums where infected individuals directly engage relevant state and non-state actors on challenges facing them and with positive feedback. They held the belief that, during such stakeholder forums, they can directly communicate their needs to HIV/AIDS policy makers and programmers, rather than the current practice where health workers who may not self-identify with their challenges represent them.

> We do not know those people at the top that we need to meet, that is my own problem. If we know those people we need to speak to; those in government and not the NGOs. Let the government call a meeting. Secondly, we should be brought in contact with the government. If they do this, we can tell the government our problems. Let them hear the problems from the horse's mouth and then we will see if they would proffer solutions to our problems. If they don't, HIV transmission will continue to increase through infected individuals, even those who know they are positive.—[Translated] HIV-seropositive woman

The underlying narrative is that HIV-seropositive women are rarely called for participation in HIV/AIDS programs and seminars that evaluate and discuss their response to interventions. In lieu, patients' complaints are channeled to NGOs by health workers. Reportedly, however, the Erhoike health center took initiatives to include HIV-infected individuals in the overall treatment process. The current structure of the Courage HIV/AIDS support group where leadership now constitutes women living with HIV is one outcome of this initiative. The aim has been to improve the experiences of HIV patients and provide a safe space where they can seek counsel from others who are also living with the virus. Prior to this, local health workers doubled as adherence counselors and facilitators of the support group.

Still, as the women argued, there is room for greater inclusion for HIV-seropositive women beyond the health facility, especially in the broader process and planning of interventions. To be sure, women continued to assert their need for more active involvement and meaningful participation in HIV/AIDS interventions.

HIV/AIDS support groups have become symbols of micro-therapeutic spaces within the larger HIV/AIDS landscape, given their ability not only to transform marginalized unhealthy subjects to empowered and healthy bodies but also to build more competent HIV/AIDS communities. In practice, HIV/AIDS support groups form the missing social link between pure biomedical treatment regimens and HIV/AIDS sufferers. For policy and planning purposes, local health support groups represent one of the ways that non-biomedical resources can be integrated into health care. For health scholars, support groups offer some insights into the kind of comprehensive healthcare package that is often touted as ideal.

Due to the transformative power of HIV/AIDS support groups, this book pushes for a recognition that provides a legitimate path to funding for support groups especially at the grassroots, to complement the work of state and non-state actors in HIV treatment efforts.

NOTES

1. Also see Chris Lyttleton, "Fleeing the Fire: Transformation and Gendered Belonging in Thai HIV/AIDS Support Groups," *Medical Anthropology: Cross Cultural Studies in Health and Illness* 23, no. 1 (2004): 6–7, https://doi/10.1080/01459740490275995; Vikas Paudel and Kedar P. Baral, "Women Living with HIV/AIDS (WLHA), Battling Stigma, Discrimination and Denial and the Role of Support Groups as a Coping Strategy: A Review of Literature," *Reproductive Health* 12, no. 53 (2015): 9–10, https://doi/10.1186/s12978-015-0032-9.

2. See "Network of People Living with HIV and AIDS in Nigeria (NEPWHAN)," About Us, Network of People Living with HIV/AIDS in Nigeria, accessed February 15, 2019, http://nepwhan.net/?page=About-Us.

3. GNP+, *HIV Leadership through Accountability Programme: GNP+, NEPWHAN. PLHIV Stigma Index Nigeria Country Assessment* (Amsterdam: GNP+, 2011), 16, http://www.stigmaindex.org/sites/default/files/reports/Nigeria%20StigmaIndex%20final_HighRs.pdf.

4. Ibid., 16–17; Network of People Living with HIV/AIDS in Nigeria, "Network of People Living with HIV and AIDS in Nigeria (NEPWHAN)."

5. Network of People Living with HIV/AIDS in Nigeria, *HIV and AIDS Work Place Policy* (Abuja: Network of People Living with HIV/AIDS in Nigerian, 2013), 4, http://nepwhan.net/assets/policy_HIV_Work_Place_Policy_June_2013.pdf; Network of People Living with HIV/AIDS in Nigeria, *Financial Policy and Procedural Manual* (Abuja: Network of People Living with HIV/AIDS in Nigerian, 2013), 11.

6. Ian Hodgson, "Empathy, Inclusion and Enclaves: The Culture of Care of People with HIV/AIDS and Nursing Implications," *Issues and Innovations in Nursing Practice* 55, no. 3 (2006): 286, https://doi/10.1111/j.1365-2648.2006.03913.x.

Chapter 8

Structuring and Stricturing Individual Coping Strategies

The previous chapter discussed HIV/AIDS support groups as the most common but organized coping mechanism for HIV-seropositive women who are confronted with the everyday ills and challenges of treatment. This chapter continues the discourse on the ways that HIV-seropositive women negotiate treatment constraints but with a focus on individualized coping mechanisms. It is a follow-up to a claim made in the preceding chapter that the reality of structural constraints to women's treatment does not eliminate personal will and effort to negotiate them. Another crucial claim made in the preceding chapter is that actual tangible resources that accrue from current HIV/AIDS interventions do not always address the treatment needs of HIV-seropositive women.

These claims segue into one of two central arguments I make in this chapter, which is that the disconnect between HIV/AIDS intervention resources and women's treatment needs mandates women to make *irrational* choices that are not only detrimental to their individual health but counterproductive to public health goals. Too often, women's choices in the quest for alternative resources may not represent logical decisions that might be assimilated under ideal circumstances but they become rational for individuals operating within a realm of restricted resources and scarce opportunities. This chapter also highlights the role of institutions and a culture that continues to place the burden of infection on individuals. It considers these factors as fundamental to regulating personal agency in negotiating treatment constraints and the rationalization of choices adopted to cope with living with HIV.

The second cardinal argument I make in this chapter is that individual negotiation of treatment constraints should not be conflated with a successful self-management as these women do not operate from a position of control, power, and absolute choice. Although the HIV-seropositive women understudied resisted treatment challenges in multiple ways, these women are not the utility-maximizing economic agents or the fully responsibilized biocitizens imagined in accounts of neoliberal and advanced liberal health citizenship.[1] Rather, using a variety of available strategies, they contest the challenges they face from a position of vulnerability, within an all-too-limited range of choices while developing resilience to survive, especially unfavorable conditions. Most of these strategies are also not sustainable in the long term because they are individualized rather than as a result of structural changes and improvements. It is also important to note that strategies deployed varied from woman to woman, depending on her particular situation. The coping mechanisms outlined in what follows are, therefore, not universally applicable to all women living with HIV.

A notion among institutional stakeholders is that infected individuals are the architects of their misfortune, rather than victims of structural violence. To explain why this critique matters, I explore how institutional irresponsibility and the overexaggeration of individual agency function as a relay of the blame-the-victim culture associated with HIV/AIDS, in many social contexts. In simple terms, this is a culture that places the fault of infection at the level of the individual. The misconstruction of HIV/AIDS transmission as individualized not only obscures its structural underpinnings, but it also minimizes or absolves institutions of their obligation to resolve the concomitant challenges while transferring the burden of care to sufferers, thus, exacerbating vulnerabilities.

On the other hand, HIV-seropositive women constructed societal victimization and blame of HIV individuals as borne out of the exceptional nature of HIV/AIDS. They demonstrated this claim through two parallel discourses: HIV/AIDS exceptionalism is beneficial because it attracts adequate attention to curtail the epidemic but inimical to the well-being of infected individuals because its exceptionality has sustained the prejudices around it. Women's accounts demonstrate that exceptionalism does not only lie in the abstract but it is also a lived experience given the ways that HIV-infected bodies are socially marked and treated differently as the virus continues to gain exceptionalism through negative media rhetoric that foster fear and stigma around infected persons. As usual, women's narratives not only help to provide context-specific dimensions to global debates, they provide on the ground insights into how some of these concepts are lived and experienced in real time. Their narratives also reemphasize the need to always make sense of universal and abstract concepts from local perspectives and concrete experiences.

INDIVIDUALIZED COPING STRATEGIES

One of the broader implications of the provision of biomedical treatment regimens without social buffers is that the responsibility to negotiate attendant challenges is vested in the individual already burdened with the vulnerabilities of infection.

Religion is a significant coping pathway for women living with HIV. Many HIV-seropositive women expressed belief in a Supreme Being that grants grace and internal strength to overcome circumstances beyond the control of mere mortals, especially in this context where some of the women described HIV/AIDS as a "wicked spirit" and their infection as "bad luck." With such spiritual affiliations, it is no wonder that many of the seropositive women sought religion to cope with the infection, and sometimes, as permanent solutions for treatment and cure.

As have been established in previous chapters, religion is core to the Nigerian society. A survey conducted by the British Broadcasting Corporation showed that Nigeria was the most engaged society in religious activities compared to other countries surveyed.[2] Expectedly, just as religion defines the values of many Nigerians, it also defines the ways that individuals seek solution to life's problems, including issues around health. The intersection of faith and HIV/AIDS underscored in women's coping strategies is a connection that has also been confirmed by similar studies in other sub-Saharan African contexts.[3] It is also one that has been acknowledged by the World Health Organization (WHO), which confirmed the need for more research into this area, given that the intersections of religion, culture, and health are still underexplored, particularly in HIV/AIDS research.[4]

Like HIV/AIDS support groups, organized religion serves as therapeutic spaces and sites of solace for many HIV-seropositive women but religious faith and belief come with particular implications for access and adherence to treatment. At the Erhoike health center, both health workers and HIV-seropositive women reported multiple cases of deaths among infected patients who discontinued treatment due to faith-based messages by religious leaders who declared them healed from HIV/AIDS. But like a female health worker narrated, poverty and education are central to how seropositive women respond to religious messaging.

> Little balancing [help or support] in the sense that they [HIV patients] can afford money to move [around]; they can eat well and they are little more exposed [so] there are no religious characteristics behind it. Some people, religious characteristics are affecting them. They will take it that God will heal me, and at the end when their situation has started deteriorating so much, they will come out again to say, treat me but that time, "water has already passed garri" [the last phrase which is Pidgin English means that "it is already too late"], that is it.—Community health worker

This excerpt depicts two categories of women. The first category is infected women who are able to manage their seropositivity because they are socially and economically empowered to do so, and, therefore, they need little to no external support. These women are not only educated so they are able to make informed decisions, but they are also able to mobilize relevant resources to adjust and cope with their new status. Religion, although may be significant to this category of women, is not pursued primarily as a coping mechanism. The second category is poor and less educated women, who rely on religion, in the absence of real and tangible alternatives to manage and cope with their seropositivity. In some instances, these women abandon ARV treatment to seek spiritual cure. When a cure does not materialize, they return to treatment but as the healthcare worker narrated, many return in a diseased state when conventional treatment is no longer possible. Among poor infected women, religious spaces are also perceived as sites to mobilize and accumulate psychosocial and material resources.

> We do not want to die now because we still love life so we continue to struggle [to live], we will struggle. It is by God's grace, and may be church [that we survive]. Like me, my church knows my status. I opened up to them, my children, everybody knows my status. So if I do not even have money, I can say "Daddy" [referring to and means "the church head or pastor"], I want to go and pick up my drugs. I even use my situation as an avenue to collect money from the church and my family because I consider myself important to them, and because I have also been good to them. So when this kind of a thing [infection] happened to me, they cannot abandon me, especially now that I am HIV-positive.—[Translated] HIV-seropositive woman

As previous analysis has established, women find disclosure difficult because of fear of real or anticipated consequences. Although social and economic security, and other perceived incentives are important motivations for disclosure, nondisclosure occurs where perceived risks outweigh perceived gains. As in the case of this woman, HIV-infected women may disclose their seropositivity to spouses, partners, family, friends, or organized groups like the church and other local support groups when there are benefits to be gained from the process, especially in coping with the virus.

The intersection of religion and HIV/AIDS thus necessitates a more effective collaboration between faith-based organizations (FBOs) and HIV/AIDS intervention efforts. Although FBOs in Nigeria have a long history of collaboration with HIV/AIDS coordinating and implementing partners, most of it has been inclined toward preventive efforts.[5] Only recently is HIV/AIDS research beginning to recognize the role of FBOs in sabotaging treatment efforts due to faith-based messaging that sometimes encourage infected individuals to abandon ARV treatment for spiritual healing.[6] It is pertinent, therefore, not to designate FBOs as just collaborators in HIV/AIDS preventive programs but their partnership should make for more meaningful involvement in treatment initiatives through the expansion of ongoing dialogues with FBOs and the development of their capacity to deliver care through appropriate messaging.

In what may be regarded as an *illogical* behavior yet engaged as a coping strategy to living with HIV, sex is reported to be sometimes commercialized among HIV-infected women to solicit for financial and material gains to meet the cost of treatment, nutrition, and other living expenses. From women's stories, HIV seropositivity does not stop indiscriminate sexual behavior but may reinforce it because seropositivity brings on new forms of marginalization. Thus, infected women, with the additional burden to care for their bodies seek ways to accumulate necessary capital even if this involves sexual practices that are inimical to their health and wellbeing. The following is the voice of one such woman who is a single parent with four children to cater to but without a sustainable means of livelihood. She had opted for what she considered her best course of action, given her available options at the time.

> For me, the truth is, before I met this man who wanted to marry me, I had three to four boyfriends that paid me so much money. I did not use condom and I could not use condom because they are rich men. And even if I had told them [I had HIV], they would not have believed me. [This continued] until last year when I met this man that promised me marriage. [He was] the kind of man that I had really prayed for [and] God brought him. So because of this man, I had to quit from all those people [the other boyfriends] and concentrate on him [alone].—HIV-seropositive woman

As a cultural trend in Nigeria, many men abhor the use of condoms during sexual intercourse because of popular beliefs, for example, that condoms as protective barriers limit sexual pleasure for men—a trend reified by a HIV-seropositive man in the support group meeting I attended at the Erhoike health center. He justified his lack of condom use during sexual intercourse with uninfected partners (who are also unaware of his seropositivity) with the argument that the risk of transmitting the virus to his partners was low because his viral load had diminished. Although this proposition is based on scientific evidence that with consistent uptake of ARVs, HIV becomes undetectable in the blood and other fluids, and therefore, dormant,[7] a high level of adherence is needed and with constant medical visits to monitor viral loads to ensure that the virus remains inactive.[8] In this state, transmission of the virus to an uninfected partner is eliminated.[9] What was not clear, however, was if this HIV-infected man had been medically certified to engage in sexual intercourse without condom or if his stance was purely presumptuous. Given the pleasure memes around non-condom use during sexual activity, unprotected sex is therefore negotiated at a higher cost among commercial sex workers or *quid pro quo* relationships where sex and money are intentionally bartered, as the above narrative illustrates.

Implicit in women's accounts was an astute sense and awareness that some of the strategies they deployed to cope with living with the virus would not be their choices if they had better alternatives. To illustrate, the HIV-seropositive woman in the aforementioned narrative had gone on to quit her multiple sexual relationships when she chanced upon a better opportunity, the alternative of a lifetime monogamous relationship through marriage. Women's choices do reveal the nature of treatment needs, structural deformities, and the weaknesses of current biomedical solutions to the social aspects of treatment, which left unattended act as catalysts for social behaviors that are counterproductive to individual health and well-being, as well as HIV/AIDS mitigation efforts.

Other coping strategies reported by women include covertly redistributing and utilizing funds originally allocated to them by their partners for household expenses to procure treatment costs such as supplementary drugs and transportation to the clinic for appointments. Although these strategies may not represent ideal and acceptable negotiation practices, it stands to reason that as an essentialized trait of the human nature, distressed subjects including HIV-seropositive women under conditions of structural neglect and the intense pressure to cope, will eke out survival mechanisms to address their immediate sufferings. The argument is not that their *irrational* decisions be regarded as absolutely logical but that certain irrational behaviors become rational in a context of survival, especially where there are limited choices and alternatives. Yet HIV/AIDS research sometimes positions infected women as active agents in their response to the social challenges of the disease because of their ability to develop individual coping mechanisms.[10] But the testimonies of women in this study compel me to take a slightly different approach and perspective to this argument.

First, this sort of generalized agency flattens out individual experiences. It also extenuates the arduous conditions less-privileged and under-empowered women navigate to cope or redress their challenges to treatment. Frequently, less-privileged HIV-seropositive women do not effectively negotiate or totally subdue the barriers to treatment even though they may develop some sort of coping mechanisms as we see from their narratives. Consequently, the everyday lives of these women are constantly characterized with the struggles of living and coping with their seropositivity, along with the persistent quest to find effective ways to manage and sustain their treatment regimen.

Second, as I argue, is that the overgeneralization of individual agency especially in marginalized contexts may unintentionally absolve institutions of their obligation to manage HIV infections at a personal level while designating structural solutions as possible within individual agencies and boundaries. I also argue that absolute agency can only be assumed when women possess complete authority and free will to control and self-determine their choices through actions that are not mediated by an unequal and oppressive system. In other words, active agency is expressed when women do not act under constraining conditions but are able to effectively improve their circumstances through unrestricted opportunities for change. An issue always to be considered in the construction of active or passive agency especially in marginalized contexts is the subjectivity of women's choices, that is, if a particular choice would be made if there were better options and if selected choices would remain constant even under improved personal conditions. If this is not in the affirmative, then we may not actively construct actions taken under marginal conditions as an expression of active or absolute agency, and stand the risk of misconstructing marginalized and structurally conditioned subjects as having the power to control and transform their circumstances just because they survived. Understanding the diversity of ways HIV-seropositive women address treatment challenges and the degree to which they improvise personal solutions to their predicament also enable us to assess their urgent need for solutions that produce better health outcomes for them. Knowledge of these choices also helps to situate coping with HIV, within the broader intercourse of individual agency and institutional obligation.

In the following section, I expose some of the factors that promote the exaggeration of personal agency, how these confer HIV-seropositive women with an assumed power for change and also position them as their own change agents, while diminishing institutional obligations.

THE CULTURE OF BLAME

We can theorize some possible reasons why undue responsibility is conferred on HIV-infected subjects. Given that a major transmission of HIV is through heterosexual relations especially in the sub-Saharan African context, HIV/AIDS-infected individuals are constructed as mostly responsible for their infection. Relatedly, the construction of risky populations at the onset of the epidemic not only created an *othering* process such that these populations were defined as vector transmitters, but it also produced a culture of blame where women, in particular, were most implicated.[11] An outcome of this social misconstruction is the perception that HIV-infected individuals must assume responsibility in the management of their infection and diseased states whether or not they are capable. This narrative held true among some policy stakeholders, health workers, as well as HIV-seropositive women. The latter, although did not explicitly blame themselves for their infection, their responses revealed that they recognized the link between individualized blame and responsibility.

Based on health workers' narratives, HIV-seropositive women are not always regarded as victims of harmful circumstances but as active perpetrators in their own infections. The widespread belief that HIV transmission

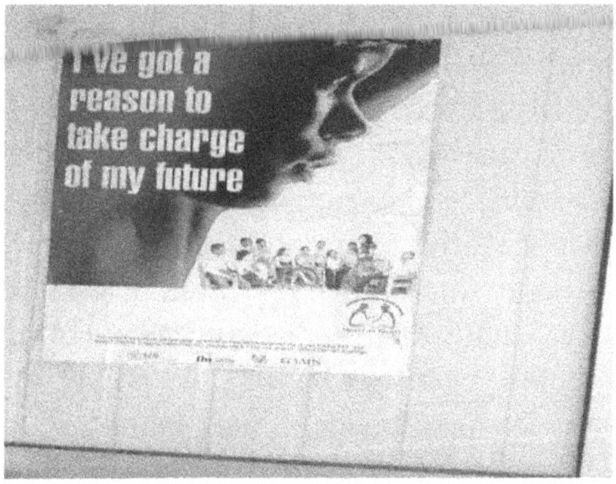

Figure 8.1 Poster transmitting a message of individual responsibility.
Source: Author, personal photography.

is primarily through sexual behavior produces moral judgments that blame infection directly on the individual, and thus, the need for such individuals to also take personal responsibility for the management of their infection. Sometimes, this moral theory provokes a lack of sympathy and empathy from health workers and the society, in general, and reportedly creates both societal- and facility-based stigma toward infected individuals who are blamed for their seropositivity. HIV/AIDS organizations are also complicit in individualizing responsibility through their messaging, as seen on this poster with the face of a female (see Figure 8.1), on the building of the Courage HIV/AIDS support group, at the Erhoike health center.

This poster captures a typical HIV/AIDS message where women are charged to take responsibility for their future. Like Caroline Faria's study of gendering responsibility in HIV/AIDS prevention and mitigation in Ghana, blame and responsibility for HIV/AIDS in the sub-Saharan African context usually bear the face of women.[12] Whether intentional or not, whether literal or figuratively, such messages and rhetoric reinforce individualized modes of health management while minimizing institutional obligation. This is not to claim that infected individuals have no responsibility toward their health citizenship, rather, HIV/AIDS messages that mostly underscore the role of individuals can undermine individual rights to hold institutions accountable for their welfare. Interestingly, HIV-seropositive women are beginning to accept these discourses of blame and individual responsibility. Women's narratives revealed a pattern where they alternated between absolving relevant institutions of their obligations and invoking personal responsibility for their health management, given institutional failures.

> To me and other people, their weakness, they [referring to HIV/AIDS institutions: NGOs and state agencies] just come and talk; they do not do what they

> say, that is the truth. They don't do what they say, they just come, talk so long as they are able to get their agenda [which are] the minutes of whatever meeting they hold [and] photographs because they have their report to submit to whoever they collected that money from. So as long as they have their reports, they are okay. They don't do what they say and it is not right. I would say [it is] because we are the ones suffering it [HIV], although they are not the ones that put us in this condition.—HIV-seropositive woman and support group leader

As we see in the preceding narrative, this HIV-seropositive woman indicts HIV/AIDS organizations as uncaring because they are perceived to execute an organizational-based agenda that precludes the interests of HIV-infected individuals. Yet she claims that these institutions cannot be held accountable because they are not responsible for the plight of infected individuals. While this claim may be somewhat true in that HIV/AIDS management must operate at multiple scales, and as a matter of shared responsibility between institutions and individuals, women's conflation of rights with privilege is problematic. The popular notion expressed among some of the women that HIV/AIDS interventions are a privilege and not an entitlement is not only flawed, but, in a context where victims of HIV transmission are constantly remarginalized and saddled with most of the responsibility of care, this is also not totally unexpected. For example, the following excerpt depicts situations where patients have been mostly saddled with the responsibility of care because HIV/AIDS institutions fall short of providing a comprehensive care package for infected individuals.

> We try to counsel them; that is what we do. We try to counsel them and we leave them to their fate.—Community health worker

Given institutional failures, women are abandoned where rudimentary counseling fails to address the challenges of living with HIV. The notion of shared responsibility should, therefore, not preclude an objective assessment of women's capabilities to redress some of these barriers, especially poor women. Similarly, it should also not excuse corporate inaction by both NGOs and state agencies as some of the women and health workers have done. It is irrational to assume that individuals who could not protect themselves from being infected and diseased because of their marginalities can suddenly confront the challenges of their new health status under the same conditions. These sorts of flawed constructions are sure to promote a *laissez-faire* attitude and institutional irresponsibility, such that institutions do not fully deliver on their duties to their citizens, especially the vulnerable ones.

In citing one of the barriers to treatment access and adherence, a majority of the HIV-seropositive women implicated the payment of user fees for the mandatory multivitamins and antibiotics for HIV/AIDS opportunistic infections. They claimed that it was already difficult sourcing for funds for transportation to the clinic but worse so, when they have to pay additional money for the supplementary drugs.

> *HPW1:* It affects. Sometimes, you can finish your drugs and you don't have the money for transportation to come pick up another set, let alone have the small money you need to drop [at the hospital]. . . . it makes one to skip taking the drugs sometimes.
>
> *EB:* Which small money are you referring to?
>
> *HPW3:* Yes, maybe like when they [we] fall sick, maybe you are having like typhoid or malaria, they [we] will have to buy drugs, once they [we] don't have the money to buy the drugs and you know, we living with this virus, we are easily affected with any kind of illness because our immune system is no longer as strong as it used to be so some can't even afford those drugs the doctor has written for them. So it is really difficult for them [us] to get the drugs since the money is not there. And even some of these multivitamins that we do buy from the hospital, not everybody [can afford it], some are pre-ART patients and these pre-ART patients, they don't take the real HIV drugs, what they take is just these multivitamins [like] septrin and there is a blood capsule; that is what they take because their CD4 is still very high so they will have to buy their drugs [the multivitamins which are not free unlike the ARVs].
>
> *EB:* So they will have to buy those ones?
>
> *HPW3:* Yes, they are buying their drug [multivitamins] . . . [but] not everyone has money to buy it and even we that are on ART, we still have to buy those same drugs also.

In contrast, some of the health workers narrated that the charge of user fees for supplementary drugs and other requirements of treatment like adequate nutrition should be a responsibility that HIV-seropositive women should be able to bear given the free provision of ARVs, as shown below. This narrative continues to underscore the ways that health workers exaggerate women's agencies and responsibilities in the management of their seropositivity.

> Well, government from what I can say, they have tried. The NGOs have tried, it is not easy to provide those drugs [ARVs] because if you say, you [patients] are going to buy those drugs, "Nigeria go die finish" [translated directly from Pidgin English means "many HIV-seropositive Nigerians will die"]. . . . If they [relevant institutions] can provide drugs, they [women] should be able to feed themselves to take the drugs.—Community health worker

While this argument may sound logical, the ability of individuals to afford small user fees and satisfy other requirements for treatment varies greatly by individual social locations and economic class. Women's responses also validate existing research evidence that user fees for health care, no matter how small, can act as a barrier to health service access especially for the very poor.[13]

CONSTRUCTING HIV/AIDS EXCEPTIONALISM FROM THE *OTHER* SIDE

The lethality and threat of HIV/AIDS to global biosecurity have, over time, culminated in an intense and expanded global-local response through donor funding, research, and scholarship.[14] This exceptional response and privileging of HIV/AIDS funding relative to other diseases is popularly referenced in scholarly texts as HIV/AIDS exceptionalism.[15] Two types of HIV/AIDS exceptionalism are described in the scholarship.[16] One in the early phase of the epidemic defined by the initial response from the West to contain what was an impending viral pandemic.[17] The second type of exceptionalism emerged from the overwhelming global response to HIV/AIDS through huge financial allocations but one that has produced an outcry from public health practitioners in other communicable infections as well as critical debates on the need to normalize the epidemic.[18]

Some of these global contestations were also reenacted in women's narratives as they inadvertently weighed in on the ways that they have been affected by the exceptionality of the disease as they responded to questions on perceptions and experiences of HIV/AIDS interventions. The aim of this section is not to explore the exceptionality debate but to draw attention to its alternative framings from the standpoint of the population most impacted, based on how women personally experience the exceptionalism of HIV/AIDS. Local perspectives based on the experiences of HIV-seropositive women illuminate the multiple ways that HIV/AIDS exceptionalism can be redefined to shape future policy considerations and actions.

Among women living with HIV, the language of exceptionalism was deployed and interpreted somewhat different from common usage in the scholarship. Like classic HIV/AIDS exceptionalism definitions, HIV-seropositive women constructed this concept in terms of the huge policy response to the epidemic but foregrounded the associated social outcomes and impact of exceptionalism on everyday life. HIV women were critical of the outcomes and current impact of interventions, especially, given the massive global policy attention the epidemic has received. They argued that efforts were incommensurate to impact mostly because there is still no cure, which is expected to demystify and normalize the epidemic. Women believed that this lack of a cure to HIV/AIDS, in addition to the extensive global and local publicity around the epidemic, has climaxed into fear and stigma rather than normalization because of lack of awareness and negative messaging reinforced by the electronic and print media.[19]

> There is a place in Warri . . . they placed this big signboard, "HIV kills." So that is bad publicity that people give to HIV. That is why people are still running away from us but if you can provide the correct information, everybody will know the real nature of HIV. People should be sensitized from community to community, radio, television, newspapers, books; just make sure that the information is spread the way the virus spreads so that if we just spread the information like that, we will see that this discrimination will be reduced. That big signboard of HIV kills, it scares people away.—HIV-seropositive woman

HIV-seropositive women opined that public health awareness campaigns aimed at improving knowledge about the epidemic sometimes served to heighten fear and stigma because some of the messages have been poorly coded with wrong and haphazard information about the pathologies of the virus. Ultimately, the resultant fear and stigma discourage testing, identification of new cases, and status disclosure. This type of exceptionalism that is borne out of huge publicity yet with a lack of awareness, the women claimed, is inimical to HIV/AIDS gaining a normalized status like other infectious diseases.

> Everybody in the world knows what malaria is and what it is not. If I have malaria, I can go to my husband and say, Honey, I went to the doctor today and I was told I have malaria. It is very easy to say I am sick of malaria and my husband will not be angry but . . . once anybody just hears the mention of HIV/AIDS, they will move away from you because of lack of awareness.—[Translated] HIV-seropositive woman

According to women's claims, HIV/AIDS exceptionalism is defined by paradoxes. While there is so much publicity around the virus, lots of myths and ignorance remain because of the ways the epidemic has been publicized. Women in their own voices have experienced the impacts of HIV/AIDS exceptionalism in very personal ways, for example, stigma, not only as a function of a lack of awareness but as a function of negative publicity and rhetoric.

Different pathways to the normalization of diseases are documented in the literature and significant among them is the availability of drugs or treatment.[20] But too often, recommendations of disease normalizations are based on Western or universal premises that elide local and cultural contexts that may produce particular prejudices, thus, making normalization impossible in these contexts.

The meanings and interpretations that HIV-seropositive women assigned to the concepts of exceptionalism and normalization were through their direct and personal experiences which are embedded within their local context. Women's interpretations of HIV/AIDS exceptionalism are localized, departing from global meanings of exceptionalism that are mostly constitutive of the lethality of this disease and its massive global funding machinery. While some of these global meanings are reflected in HIV-seropositive women's interpretations of HIV/AIDS exceptionalism, their personal experiences proffer insights into the contextual implications of exceptionalism. For example, HIV-seropositive women argued for AIDS normalization but not in the conventional forms argued by public health practitioners who call for less funding and the redistribution of funds to other diseases. While the women applauded the huge funds allocated for HIV/AIDS interventions in which they are beneficiaries, they argued that funds should also be appropriately channeled to eliminate the negative constructions associated with the virus. For HIV-seropositive women, AIDS normalization is when the disease is less stigmatized and no longer perceived as a death threat, and when sufferers are no longer socially criminalized.

HIV/AIDS exceptionalism, although a global construct, is experienced locally and in ways that are spatially contingent. HIV-seropositive women's experiences and interpretations also illuminate the paradox of HIV/AIDS exceptionalism, in that its exceptionality has attracted not only huge positive benefits in terms of intervention resources but also a high level of stigma. Women's experiences also signal the relevance of scale and the application of local perspectives to drive and resolve global debates, as well as global decision-making.

The nature of coping strategies and the categories of women that deploy them consistently reveal differences among women's choices and reestablish the need for policy and programs to target women as a heterogeneous group of individuals with disparate needs. They also reveal that women enact different levels of agency in negotiating and coping with the challenges of treatment because individual social locations impact individual experiences and, in this case, ability to negotiate seropositivity.

This chapter reiterates that quick-fix behavioral strategies and other forms of extemporized coping mechanisms cannot function in lieu of structural mechanisms to address the challenges of HIV-seropositive women, with individualized coping strategies that imply that infected women must take personal responsibility for their care in the absence of structural solutions. Likewise, deploying personal strategies for structural problems is not sustainable in the long haul as most of these strategies are contingent and temporary solutions, in that they take the form of everyday exigencies quickly deployed for immediate respite. The implication is that these survival tactics become entrenched in the everyday lives of women as they are continuously recycled to negotiate treatment challenges on a regular basis, thereby, launching women into an endless and vicious circle of health and social tragedy.

NOTES

1. See Nikolas Rose, "The Politics of Life Itself," *Theory, Culture and Society* 18, no. 6 (December 2001).

2. "Nigeria Leads in Religious Belief," *British Broadcasting Corporation News*, last modified February 26, 2004, http://news.bbc.co.uk/2/hi/programmes/wtwtgod/3490490.stm.

3. See O. Oluduro, "The Role of Religious Leaders in Curbing the Spread of HIV/AIDS in Nigeria," *Potchefstroom Electronic Law Journal* 13, no. 3 (2010); Omobolaji O. Olarinmoye, "Faith-Based Organizations and Development: Prospects and Constraints," *Transformation: An International Journal of Holistic Mission Studies* 29, no. 1 (2012).

4. "Faith-Based Organizations Play a Major Role in HIV/AIDS Care and Treatment in Sub-Saharan Africa," World Health Organization, last modified February 8, 2007, http://www.who.int/mediacentre/news/notes/2007/np05/en/.

5. For example, see Jude Aguwa, "Religion and HIV/AIDS Prevention in Nigeria," *Cross Currents* (2010); Oluduro, "The Role of Religious Leaders in Curbing the Spread of HIV/AIDS in Nigeria."

6. World Health Organization, "Faith-Based Organizations."

7. "Viral Suppression for HIV Treatment Success and Prevention of Sexual Transmission of HIV," HIV/AIDS, World Health Organization, accessed February 19, 2019, https://www.who.int/hiv/mediacentre/news/viral-supression-hiv-transmission/en/.

8. Camille Arkell and Mallory Harrigan, "HIV Treatment and an Undetectable Viral Load to Prevent HIV Transmission," *CATIE*, last modified 2018, https://www.catie.ca/en/fact-sheets/transmission/hiv-viral-load-hiv-treatment-and-sexual-hiv-transmission.

9. World Health Organization, "Viral Suppression for HIV Treatment Success and Prevention of Sexual Transmission of HIV."

10. For example, see Pranee Liamputtong, Niphattra Haritavorn, and Niyada Kiatying-Angsulee, "HIV and AIDS, Stigma and AIDS Support Groups: Perspectives from Women Living with HIV and AIDS in Central Thailand," *Social Science and Medicine* (2009), https://doi.org/10.1016/j.socscimed.2009.05.040.

11. For example, see Phillip Setel, *A Plague of Paradoxes: AIDS, Culture and Demography in Northern Tanzania* (Chicago: University of Chicago Press, 2000), 211.

12. See Caroline Faria, "Privileging Prevention, Gender Responsibility: An Analysis of the Ghanaian Campaign against AIDS," *Social and Cultural Geography* 9, no. 1 (February 2008), https://doi.org/10.1080/14649360701789584.

13. See Isaac A. O. Odeyemi and John Nixon, "Assessing Equity in Health Care through the National Health Insurance Schemes of Nigeria and Ghana: A Review-Based Comparative Analysis," *International Journal for Equity in Health* 12, no. 9 (2013): 2.

14. William A. Fisher, Taylor Kohut, and Jeffrey D. Fisher, "AIDS Exceptionalism: On the Social Psychology of HIV Prevention Research," *Social Issues Policy Review* 3, no. 1 (December 2009): 6, https://doi.org/10.1111/j.1751-2409.2009.01010.x.

15. See Ronald Bayer, "Public Health Policy and the AIDS Epidemic: An End to HIV Exceptionalism?" *New England Journal of Medicine* 324, no. 21 (1991), where the term HIV Exceptionalism first appeared. Also see Gerald M. Oppenheimer and Ronald Bayer, "The Rise and Fall of AIDS Exceptionalism," *American Medical Association Journal of Ethics* 11, no. 12 (2009): 988.

16. Lisa Forman, "Global AIDS Funding and the Re-Emergence of AIDS 'Exceptionalism'," *Social Medicine* 6, no. 1 (2011): 45–48. Also see Julia H. Smith and Alan Whiteside, "Exceptional Epidemics: AIDS Still Deserves a Global Response," *Globalization and Health* 5, no. 15 (2009).

17. Ibid., 1.

18. Ibid., 2.

19. See Herek et al., "Workshop Report: AIDS and Stigma: A Conceptual Framework and Research Agenda," *AIDS and Public Policy Journal* 13, no. 1 (Spring 1998): 43.

20. See Rolf Rosenbrock et al., "The Normalization of AIDS in Western European Countries," *Social Science and Medicine* 50 (2000).

Part 3

MODELS OF INTERVENTIONS

Chapter 9

Beyond the Rhetoric of Gender Mainstreaming

In theory, there is no difference between theory and practice. But in practice, there is.

—Jan L. A. van de Snepscheut[1]

For those of us committed to effecting practical change through research, a major challenge and continuous point of tension in positively transforming the lives of the subjects and spaces that we so enthusiastically study is the translation of theory into practice. The theorizing of real-life issues for the sole purpose of producing academic knowledge becomes inadequate when we recognize the need for knowledge to transform conceptual spaces through concrete actions, in order to positively alter the lives of people around which we produce knowledge. But it is at the point where we attempt to leap beyond the boundaries of theory that we face the multifaceted and real-world complexities that drive a wedge between theory and practice. The tension between theory and practice is no different from that experienced within development spaces where effectively translating policy into concrete actions seems to be a huge challenge.[2]

This chapter responds to a central issue that frames this book, which is the attempt to move the theory of gender mainstreaming beyond the rhetoric of a transformative ideology to actually engendering social justice and progressive change for women through effective development practices. The arguments in this chapter build on a fundamental premise that is based on the results of a critical discourse analysis of HIV/AIDS policy texts, detailed in chapter 2 of this book, which is that the mainstreaming of gender in Nigerian HIV/AIDS policies is problematic and incoherent, given the ideological contradictions in the ways that gender is framed across policy plans. Similarly, an analysis of in-depth interviews with public and private sector HIV/AIDS policy stakeholders (hereafter, referred to as policy stakeholders), which forms the crux of this chapter, confirms this trend.[3] The chapter contributes to ongoing global analyses around the not-so-successful implementation of gender policies in third world spaces through a two-pronged objective.

First, the chapter demonstrates using primary evidence, local factors that drive tensions between the theory and the practice of gender mainstreaming, in the Nigerian context. Central to this objective is to illustrate the ways that power may be permeated through institutional processes to oppress and disempower minority, powerless, and marginal groups like HIV-seropositive women, albeit unintentionally. Institutional blocs to gender mainstreaming in this context include poor or lack of gender mainstreaming knowledge, institutional resistance, and the lack of political will. Furthermore, policy stakeholders' narratives reveal a poor framing and interpretation of gender, and a conflict in the models of gender equity adopted, which appear to undermine the effective translation of gender mainstreaming into practice. This claim is premised on scholarly arguments that effective gender mainstreaming is contingent on how gender is framed or conceptualized.[4] Policy stakeholders' narratives, however, show that beyond the correct framing and interpretation of gender, identity politics is also an important barrier to effective gender mainstreaming in the Nigerian context.

Second, the chapter draws attention to the role of global health institutions and how their power-laden transnational relations shape local orientations of gender through the transfer of knowledge and policies from the globalizing spaces of the North to the South. Significant to this argument are the specific ways that immanent development activities of international governance systems and transnational aid networks channeled through the NGO mechanism and bi/multilateral arrangements condition the ways that global health interventions are localized and implemented.

NGOs' connections to transnational funding networks not only drive their local agenda, but they also structure the forms of knowledge integrated into interventions, including gender. As a consequence, NGOs' generic capabilities to streamline local contexts into development strategies and rework mainstream interventions in socially, culturally, and politically appropriate ways are stymied, despite recurrent notions of NGOs being grounded in local knowledge. The chapter also highlights contradictions in the ideology and adoption of the gender equity agenda among international development agencies that privilege or underprivilege gender in HIV/AIDS interventions. Similarly, the adoption of the ideology of gender mainstreaming as a priority agenda is not uniform across donor organizations within the global HIV/AIDS community. Through multiple vertical funding relationships with indigenous development practitioners, these inconsistencies are reproduced on the local landscape and create tensions in the policy and practice of gender mainstreaming. In exploring these issues, thus, the role of *context* as significant to understanding why gender mainstreaming is not effective is also underscored but context as deployed here foregrounds the embeddedness and situatedness of places under the influence of global conditions.

GENDER MAINSTREAMING

As defined by the United Nation's Economic and Social Council (ECOSOC):[5]

> Mainstreaming a gender perspective is the process of assessing the implications for women and men of any planned action, including legislation, policies or programs, in all areas and at all levels. It is a strategy for making women's as well as men's concerns and experiences an integral dimension of the design, implementation, monitoring and evaluation of policies and programs in all political, economic and societal spheres so that women and men benefit equally and inequality is not perpetuated. The ultimate goal is to achieve gender equality.

Gender mainstreaming evolved from concerns about the need to create equality for women in terms of power, opportunities, and resources. Policies that were women-focused were thus advocated for and initiated to enable women to make incremental progress and advancements toward their male counterparts.[6] These women-only or gender-specific strategies launched through the 1975 World Conference of the International Women's Year in Mexico, were later judged to have failed to provide equality for women.[7] A major reason that was cited for this failure is that existing policies and programs were too specific to women in that they did not seek to change the structures of male domination that continue to reproduce female subordination.[8] Incorporating women's interests in all policy sections and guidelines in relation to men, in what is now formally labeled as gender mainstreaming, thus emerged as a more structural solution to empowering women.[9]

Established at the Fourth United Nations World Conference on Women in Beijing, in 1995, gender mainstreaming as a global strategy became institutionalized as a tool to promote gender equality in development.[10] In 1997, the United Nation's ECOSOC established the resolution on gender mainstreaming that gender must be ensured in all aspects of an organization, as well as policies and programs in development work.[11] By doing so, an anticipated outcome has been the restructuring of processes and other systemic relations that reproduce women's socioeconomic vulnerability and disempowerment.[12] The approach of *mainstreaming* was, thus, seen as the key to institutionalizing and forwarding structural shifts toward achieving gender equality within organizations and all spheres of public and private life.[13]

Although the shift from a narrow to a generalized approach to conceptualizing gender was to challenge and undermine processes and relations that reproduce existing inequalities between men and women,[14] current failures of gender mainstreaming in many spatial contexts have led to a stream of critiques from scholars who argue that this approach has not lived up to its practical expectations.[15] For many such scholars, gender mainstreaming is an "empty signifier."[16]

Current debates reveal gender mainstreaming as a much-contested phenomenon. Perhaps, one of the most cited critiques of gender mainstreaming and a commonly referenced reason for its failure is that gender mainstreaming is often framed and deployed in a macro and top-down prescriptive manner that neglects the political, social and cultural processes that frame local gender dynamics.[17] That is, too frequently, gender mainstreaming is constructed in very problematic ways in that its framings ignore recognition and attention to context, for example, indigenous interpretations of feminism and gender equality that may contradict orthodox or universal prescriptions, with the effect that gender mainstreaming practice becomes undermined.[18]

Critical attention to context also means that methods and implementation of gender mainstreaming must be thoroughly interrogated through questions about process, for example, the ways that gender is inserted into interventions to challenge and rework structures that reproduce inequalities.[19] Questions around the appropriate conceptualization of gender mainstreaming must be asked and critical attention must also be paid to the methods deployed to provide functionality to gender mainstreaming in development practice.[20] Yet, as a method and practice, gender mainstreaming is argued to lack rigor, given the little attention it pays to how inequality is reproduced through local and institutional processes.[21] For example, a study conducted on drought policy in Australia had revealed flaws in the implementation of gender mainstreaming in rural development policies in Europe.[22] Attempts at gender mainstreaming had been fragmented, at best providing temporary succor for women through empowerment programs that tended to leave women stranded because they were not geared to engender women's autonomy; rather, keep them solely dependent on empowerment programs.

Methodologically, gender mainstreaming has been criticized as overly superficial because it provides a vague approach to implementation.[23] Besides, its supposedly superficial nature and lack of clear implementation strategies easily lend it to multiple interpretations, which may reproduce inequalities among populations it has been designed to empower.[24] Multiple documentations of failure, especially in implementation, have led many scholars to argue that gender mainstreaming is easier to theorize but harder to translate into concrete activities that meet stated goals.[25]

Also critical to the debate on the context of gender mainstreaming is that its practice underscores particular relations of power while it obscures others at the level of institutions, for example, among policy makers, and between policy makers and recipients, because gender mainstreaming is embedded within cultural struggles that intersect with identity politics.[26] In the same way, gender mainstreaming is argued to reproduce inequality through competing policy agendas that produce a bias and preference in terms of which agenda is prioritized, and otherwise, may force compatibility of agendas even where these are incongruous.[27]

Like social and cultural factors, political will is also a very important index for an effective and successful gender mainstreaming but it is lacking in many contexts as funds to engender gender-sensitive development in public health remain far-fetched.[28] As feminist scholars argue, gender visibility in policies does not necessarily translate to real improvement in the lives of women and men, if unaccompanied with the political power and material agency especially needed to transform the unequal structures that produce harmful gender norms.[29]

These many debates underpin the focus of this chapter, which interrogates and illuminates the ways that current approaches to mainstreaming gender in HIV/AIDS interventions in Nigeria may reproduce health challenges for HIV-seropositive women. Such investigation is even more pertinent, given the persistent challenges of treatment among women amid gender policy claims.

THE GENDER KNOWLEDGE GAP

Within the private and public HIV/AIDS subsectors, policy stakeholders' narratives revealed a general lack of awareness, and/or poor knowledge of gender mainstreaming. Gender mainstreaming illiteracy can be argued to be rooted in the ways that respective organizations and departments within the health sector are internally structured. Organizations are fragmented and compartmentalized by program area which make the knowledge of gender mainstreaming to be mostly concentrated among few policy stakeholders whose program areas have clear connections to gender. This treatment of gender issues as the purview of specific departments and isolated program units within organizations constitutes a gap in knowledge and implementation.

> We have a gender unit that is very separate from the [HIV] treatment unit [and] I am speaking to you for [as] someone coming from the treatment unit. I am not really aware what the gender unit [does or] what they have prepared for their gender program.—Male NGO stakeholder

In one of the two NGOs I examined, which I refer to as NGO X, there appeared to be no integrative effort to mainstream gender as a cross-cutting issue into all program areas due to internal organizational structure.[30] In the preceding quote, a key officer from NGO X stated that he was not wholly immersed in the knowledge of gender issues neither did he possess knowledge of gender mainstreaming because gender as a unit was distinct from his unit. Ironically, this was the HIV treatment and care unit. Initially, he claimed ignorance of the knowledge of gender mainstreaming even though he stated that he was familiar with the term. On explaining this concept to him, he claimed that some form of gender mainstreaming does take place in the treatment unit but this only emerged as an afterthought because the issues that typically constrain treatment uptake were recognized to have a gender dimension. Gender mainstreaming in this NGO was thus treated as an *ad hoc* solution and not an intentional practice, and driven by expediencies that field staff considered potentially detrimental to program objectives and targets.

In NGO Y, gender mainstreaming appeared to be driven by personal interest and its perceived relevance to specific program areas as a female staff indicated, and like NGO X, it was not practiced as an institutional policy that was generally integrated into all aspects of the organization and programs.

> *EB:* so what is your understanding of gender mainstreaming?
>
> *P:* oh dear, we had an orientation on gender mainstreaming but because it doesn't feature so much in lab [referring to her unit] but my personal understanding of gender mainstreaming is just having women reached, having men reached but . . . I am not really interested in gender mainstreaming as such . . . personally, it is not an area of interest for me so I don't know much about it but when the gender component started coming up within the organization, there was orientation on it and my personal reading was just a little reading, just to have an idea of what gender was all about but I knew that it was not all about sex as in male [or] female but it goes beyond to the perception about roles and responsibilities of health issues, community issues but to be frank I know little.

This stakeholder's position also raises the issue of compatibility, of gender mainstreaming with specific program areas that are perceived as essentially technical, in this instance, the HIV laboratory. Or perhaps, it is, as have been argued, a lack of clear strategies as to how the mainstreaming of gender can be implemented in such areas, an issue that does indeed question its methodological strength.

The impression of gender as a distinct entity is also prevalent in the public health sector as gender mainstreaming is designated mainly within the purview of the Gender Technical Committee (GTC) rather than horizontal across relevant parastatals and policy stakeholders.[31] Among the GTC members and other policy stakeholders knowledgeable in gender issues, there is a deep recognition of the intersectionality of HIV/AIDS; hence, a multisectoral approach has been deployed to tackle the epidemic. This approach requires cross-sectoral collaboration among different ministries such as Education, Women Affairs, Agriculture, and Transportation, among others, to address the different but related dimensions of the epidemic. The national GTC places gender at the core of this response. Yet this multisectoral response is also what undermines the smooth incorporation of gender into policy plans.

To illustrate this, there were reported instances where HIV/AIDS-related work in the FMoH was halted because some groundwork that was supposed to be provided by other ministries was not done. Similarly, HIV/AIDS parastatals and agencies that work on similar programs were not always able to effectively collaborate because they are structured independently, and with separate leadership, finance, and budgets, as explained by this female policy stakeholder. In effect, this makes a principle like gender mainstreaming which needs a seamless coordination difficult to implement.

> I will cite an example for you. You have NACA and you have NASCP, the HIV division [in the FMoH]. Then you have malaria, and then you have tuberculosis. And malaria is a program that you have a national malaria program but you don't have an agency that controls malaria. So malaria is like one program body, tuberculosis is like one program body [but] we have HIV/AIDS division [in the FMoH] and NACA [as a separate agency]. So why don't we have them as one division so that they can plan very well? For instance, [if] NACA has a meeting today, [the] HIV/AIDS division [in the FMoH] will have the same meeting that NACA just had tomorrow. So now we are doing duplicates of many things while we are under one umbrella and we are talking about gender mainstreaming? So they are still repeating the same thing and all of us are still trying to cover the same population in quote while we are doing the same thing. So what I am saying is that, putting all these programs under gender mainstreaming can help you monitor what you are doing, that is, one program [and] only one head. We can't have two directors-generals for one program [as it is for the national HIV/AIDS response] . . . there is no collaboration, we are supposed to be working [together], NACA is supposed to be multisectoral response to HIV, while NASCP for the FMoH response but NACA is doing the work of NASCP and even doing more because they have more funding than NASCP because most funding of HIV goes to NACA so making NASCP people almost like redundant.—Former gender unit desk person, FMoH

Due to the independent structures of NASCP and NACA, national policy plans on HIV/AIDS are for the most part uncoordinated and out of sync and, by implication, challenge the smooth adoption and practice of gender mainstreaming. In a wider application, this issue of health systems fragmentation, thus, illuminates it as a key barrier to gender mainstreaming efforts in Nigeria. Gender mainstreaming as a systems-wide focus and concern illustrates the problems with verticalized interventions which fragment local health systems through separate accounting systems for the specific intervention in question, as well as a separate reporting structure to local stakeholders and international donors.[32] Verticalized interventions produce limited collaboration, duplication of efforts, wastage of scarce funding resources, and poor communication and feedback, among others. Gender mainstreaming not only illuminates the type of broader health structure that is disenabling to its successful implementation, it also reveals the much needed integrated and systems-wide approach it requires to thrive. In this context, effective gender mainstreaming is weakened by the fragmented structure of the local health system, which in large part, is influenced by international donor-funding activities.

The policy analysis also revealed that the evolution, awareness, and official adoption of gender mainstreaming across Nigeria's public health sector have not been instantaneous across parastatals. There are marked variations in the interest and knowledge of gender issues, which also shape funding priorities and budget allocations.

> [One of the] challenges, just like I told you before [is that] the gender desk could not be established. When I ceased to be the gender focus person . . . many other persons did not want to reckon with [gender] to the extent that I was asked to make some proposals so as to fund gender. Many other things will go [approved], gender will not go. So from the onset, they [policy makers] were not really interested in gender. That is one of the challenges. People at the helm of affairs, they feel gender is not one of their [problems] although the GTC see it that it is an issue and they are the [only] ones pursuing the issue of gender in the country.—Former gender unit desk person, FMoH

Evidently, the interest, urgency, and political will to address gender issues are not equally diffused across parastatals in Nigeria's public health sector. The narrative also reinforces my earlier argument that the knowledge and practice of gender mainstreaming are marginalized and isolated to units or committees, and in the national public health sector, it is the GTC. Although not referenced in the preceding narrative, a gender unit existed in the HIV/AIDS division of the FMoH, which was managed by the narrator. In 2005, however, the gender unit was dissolved when the policy official who appointed the narrator as a gender desk person was replaced by someone who was not interested in gender issues. As at the time of this interview, in December 2014, there was still no gender desk person in the HIV/AIDS division of the FMoH. The poor recognition of the importance of gender in health policy also brings with it a lack of political commitment, which is a significant challenge to successful gender mainstreaming.

POLITICS OF IDENTITY AND THE CONFLICTING MODELS OF GENDER MAINSTREAMING

Gender mainstreaming, although relatively new in Nigeria, as the policy analysis revealed, is garnering institutional attention especially among HIV/AIDS policy stakeholders due to factors that are both local and global, namely, global policy trends and existing social realities but conflicting policy discourses in the models of gender equity as well as identity politics cripple its successful implementation, in this context. Among policy stakeholders, the need to be seen as up to date with global gender equity trends in development, particularly agitations for women empowerment in the MDGs, Beijing and the Convention on the Elimination of all Forms of Discrimination Against Women (CEDAW) projects, have been cited as significant to why gender mainstreaming is garnering attention institutionally. In this sense, gender mainstreaming is adopted to showcase that local policy makers are keeping up with trends in global policy developments even though its actual practice is given little attention. Also, the age-long marginalization of women in Nigeria that recently, has been reinforced by the feminized nature of the HIV/AIDS epidemic in Nigeria (and in sub-Saharan Africa generally) has driven motivations for gender equity, particularly the need to empower women through policies and programs. But internal conflicts among policy makers, shaped by identity and gender politics, produce multiple orientations and models of gender equity. As have been argued, variabilities in the deployment of gender equity models render gender mainstreaming a contested site and also complicated in practice, especially when the differences across these models are not reconciled to form a coherent gender framework.[33]

Three models of gender equity with potentially different outcomes are identified in the gender scholarship.[34] In the sameness gender equity model, women aspire to the same equality as men and are enabled to enter into domains that continue to be dominated and controlled by men. The difference gender equity model recognizes social differences between women and men and places values on their different contributions to society. The transformative model seeks to achieve gender equity by transforming gender relations. In the analysis of policy stakeholders' narratives (including analytical reviews of policy texts), two of these three gender equity models were shown to be dominant: the sameness and transformative models. Perhaps, because gender as a construct and experience is fluid, it lends itself to diverse interpretations based on individual subjectivities, bias, and cultural context. As a result, affiliated practices like the mainstreaming of gender into policy and programs become amenable to multiple interpretations and methodological pluralism across and within diverse spatial contexts.

For the most part, policy stakeholders did not explicitly articulate a distinct model of gender equity. Rather, their narratives sometimes revealed a construction of gender equity that simultaneously engaged multiple frames. To bridge existing inequalities between men and women, there were recommendations, mostly among female policy stakeholders, of women-focused programs to empower women with access to resources like men. This women-focused model of intervention, although justified by the logic of recognition-redistribution, given women's marginalities, also appeared to be a function of identity politics.[35] For "fairness," "justice," and "equity," a female policy maker argued that current HIV/AIDS interventions should be skewed toward women because they have been long marginalized; hence, the needs of women must be privileged over men. This logic of recognition-redistribution functions by recognizing existing inequalities between men and women, and seeks to eliminate them or at least bridge the gap by redistributing resources to women.[36] In this sense, gender equity for women was conflated with sameness to men, with the argument that women like men should be positioned on the same pedestal of power and access to life's resources and opportunities.

Policy makers also invoked the transformative gender equity model with recommendations to target the relational dynamics between men and women. These multiple gender equity frames are testament to the tension and conflict among institutional actors on best strategies to achieve equality for women with interpretations of gender equality as sometimes specific to women, and at other times, integrative of both men and women. Nevertheless, the politics of identity, as it helps to perpetuate these divergent gender views, is not completely unrecognized among policy makers. Still, this recognition and the inherent complication of adopting competing gender equity models do not obviate the pursuit of a gender equality agenda that seems to serve specific gender interest among policy stakeholders, as one of them narrates.

> I remember the first meeting, the first year we had a plan, a gender mainstreaming work plan or something like that for HIV and AIDS, and I chaired that, and I was having problems with the gender committee because it is like 95 percent women and I happened to be the only [male] person. There was a time they [women] were threatening me that I was not gender sensitive [laughs] because I was defending the interests of men and all of them were defending the interest of women [laughs]; although, we know gender goes beyond men and women. . . . Even though we seem to have the theoretical meaning of gender, we seemed to understand the theoretical meaning of gender [but] when it comes to practicing it, people have different orientation as to how to really practice gender. . . . I find out that even though I have the statistics, I present the statistics most of the time about women but women are seeing gender as more of sex, female, female, female, male, male, male, but gender should be about dynamics, about relationship between the two and how this relationship predispose or make

> people vulnerable, and how do we do this? It's not just about male, male, [or] what can I do to make sure that males are represented or males have services but we need to look at the dynamics, the relationship and how this relationship has become a serious factor in the epidemic. . . . When you define it [gender], people will have correct definition but when it comes to implementation, people are divided.—Male policy stakeholder and former chair of the GTC

While the transformative model of gender equity has been touted as more sustainable because it embeds equality in social systems rather than isolates it,[37] there is little evidence that this model has been deployed as the mainstream, in the Nigerian context. In spite of the tensions among policy makers as to the correct framing of gender, gender equality was mostly rationalized within intellectual constructions that emphasized the relationality of men and women. Furthermore, in instances where the transformative approach to gender mainstreaming was articulated by policy makers, clear recommendations on practical implementation were, nevertheless, lacking. In HIV/AIDS policy texts, however, solutions to gender inequality are mostly constructed and designed as categorical or specific to women, for example, the popular prevention from mother-to-child transmission (PMTCT) program that shows little male considerations. In other words, the transformative approach to mainstreaming gender in interventions may be a fairly popular discourse among policy planners and texts but it is not always matched in practice, particularly in the type of programs that are truly gender-inclusive and aim at reworking the underlying forces that marginalize women.

Although women-only programs are directed to the needs of vulnerable women and may even empower them in the short term, they are not sustainable as they oversimplify the complexity of structures that produce inequalities (and leave them untouched) with the assumption that exclusively designed women-focused programs will erase the roots and hidden structures of inequalities in male-dominated spaces.[38] Furthermore, as I have argued in a previous chapter, in addition to breeding resistance from men, a lack of male involvement in female empowerment programs may undermine accessibility to resources supposedly redistributed through women-focused programs, especially among women who may need spousal consent to be a part of such programs.

Reportedly, gender equality is also feminized among international agencies. According to a female policy stakeholder, "a lot of partners concentrate more on women, especially the UN agencies." The feminization of gender equality, and thus the equivocation of empowerment programs with women, has met with resistance among male policy stakeholders. A female policy maker cited the public outcry among male policy makers with the establishment of the "Federal Ministry of Women Affairs." Men were reported to have felt neglected and outside the loop of gender-focused programs, and which reinforces some of the ways that institutions can embody and reproduce resistance especially to women's empowerment when gender approaches are exclusionary. A real danger, therefore, is that the practice of gender mainstreaming may become an avenue through which particular relations of power among policy actors are reperpetuated and institutionalized.

> You see, for our society, you find that the woman is actually disadvantaged in 99.9 [percent]. I don't know, I am not quoting anybody but I am just saying because if you look at everything, the woman is always more disadvantaged so you find that programs have to focus more on women. That is why there was a Ministry of Women Affairs created but overtime they [men] said, "ah, you women," you know this mentality, women "Beijing platform, they like talking about themselves" and you find out that you need to reprogram to carry along men as much as possible because they too have issues, their own issues.—Female policy stakeholder

Distrusts and divisions among men and women interest groups may turn the practice of gender mainstreaming into a site of political struggle, institutional and identity politics in policy domains, and in turn, influence how and where resources should be allocated. Local realities and struggles may, thus, reconfigure the meaning and practical application of gender mainstreaming in particular contexts. The adoption of multiple gender equity models also presents its own challenges, especially at the level of implementation. In principle, adopting both the sameness and transformative gender equity models appear complementary and also logical, given women's situational context. However, the contradictions in these different models also have the potential to manifest in a pluralism of gender programs that countervail each other in terms of practical outcomes, especially in the absence of deliberate efforts to reconcile their inherent differences. Perhaps, it is these operational difficulties that have formed the basis of critics' arguments that gender mainstreaming is a mere rhetoric if the theory of it offers more than can be feasibly and effectively practiced.[39]

GLOBAL HEALTH REGULATORY FRAMEWORKS AND THE FUNDING POLITICS OF INTERNATIONAL ORGANIZATIONS

The argument that attention to local contexts is indeed crucial to how we understand gender mainstreaming and its effectiveness is reified by the narratives of policy makers in the preceding section.[40] But the relevance of context is not exclusive to the local but extends to the global, in the ways that international organizations mediate the governance and practices of local health systems. In the Nigerian context, this is demonstrated through conflicting interests and a lack of commitment to gender issues through gender-neutral funding priorities. Institutionalized global health norms that are inimical to gender mainstreaming also misinform local understanding and practice.

Issues of donor priorities and funding as major limitations against the effective practice of gender mainstreaming are evidenced in the accounts of NGO practitioners in the private HIV/AIDS subsector. These issues speak to the general skepticism around the complex but unequal relationship that exists between NGOs as civil society organizations and the world of donor agencies cum the global political economy of development aid, and the ways they structure the forms of developmental activities that NGOs undertake. This indirect but strong influence on NGOs situatedness at the grassroots and strategies to address social problems is aptly labeled as stovepiping.[41] Stovepiping describes the nature of donor-funded interventions as mostly a reflection of the interests and concerns of the sponsors and not the recipients.[42] This is not to argue that NGOs do not have their own local mission and agenda rooted in their commitment to the needs of the population they serve but their generic non-state and for nonprofit nature usually means that they have to rely on external sources for funds to implement their agenda.[43]

Given the discourses of corruption and mismanagement of funds around public sector institutions, NGOs as non-state agents are considered as viable alternatives to mainstream national development by bi/multilateral organizations and private corporate philanthropists who seek active engagement in the international development space.[44] NGOs have, thus, been coopted into the transnational development space and in partnership with international development agencies through their need for funding—a partnership that often appears to be an alignment of development goals and a commitment to domestic priorities. Many times, this is a catch-22 situation where these global-local or local-global alliances are not always compatible with the missions and goals of NGOs. Nevertheless, much of the intentional development by NGOs is only possible because of these global-aid relations. It is within this conundrum of paradoxes and contradictions that NGOs operate and must choose whose agenda to implement, and whether to make good or not their commitment to grassroots issues. In these kinds of situations, how do NGOs respond?

Not surprising, lack of funds was repeatedly implicated as a dire challenge to the practice of gender mainstreaming across all HIV/AIDS organizations investigated for this research but mostly among NGOs. The dominant narrative among NGO stakeholders is that NGOs choose their projects based on donor-made rules guiding the allocation of funding for proposed interventions. Doing the contrary precariously places them in a situation where they are faced with the threat and possibility of exclusion and ultimately extinction from the international development landscape as this senior executive in NGO X narrated.

> The way I see it is this, if it is an environment where NGOs, [where] there is an easy access to funds for NGOs, I will say NGOs will be more independent to pursue their original mission and vision. You check most NGOs, they have their own mission and vision but they have to immediately forget that mission and vision when they are sourcing for funds and align straight with the mission and vision of their funders, so that is what is going on. Most NGOs are living from palm to hands and they have staff, so commitment is there, and they have offices they have to pay for, so when the rubber meets the ground the story changes immediately.—Male NGO stakeholder

In spite of their strong civil society roots and grassroots affiliations, the organic structure of NGOs is such that their ability to perform development on the local scene is largely contingent on the strength of their global financial ties but this can also be detrimental to local interests when aid and funding networks are opposed to specific domestic priorities, for example, gender mainstreaming. As sites of alternative and critical development, NGOs are frequently at social and political crossroads, whether to make the decision to cater to locally identified needs or to pacify donor agencies.[45] For the sustainability of their organizations, however, NGOs often prioritize the needs of donors for continued access to funds. Hence, local development efforts continue to be more rooted in the mandates of transnational development organizations than the population NGOs were originally instituted to serve.

Funds direct the nature of interventions or what components are planned for and implemented. Like the stakeholder's excerpt above indicates, NGOs may have good intentions that mirror the needs of the grassroots population and subjects of interventions but oftentimes, have to change or rearticulate their mission and vision statement to align and reflect the needs and agenda of funders. Constantly realigning their organization's mission to funders' objectives in the bidding process for donor-sponsored projects is a major way that NGOs can access funds from donors and keep their organizations afloat with respect to administrative and overhead costs. In many ways, this confirms debates in the alternative development scholarship of NGOs as not been autonomous but linked to global political economy forces of development, re-creating a form of mainstream development that may nullify the agenda and civic nature of NGOs.[46] Also, as I argue, NGOs dependencies on external aid reflect new forms of imperialism channeled through international development agencies as machineries, in contradiction to popular anti-imperialists perceptions of NGOs or NGOs as agents of alternative and critical development.[47] In this way, indigenous global health NGOs have been launched into the formal global capitalist economy as they redirect the production of health services toward the direction of capital flow.

As already established, the funding structure of NGOs can undermine commitment to programs that are gender-based if this is not a donor priority. It is important to note, however, as alluded by NGO X, that the funders they have worked with have not always outright opposed the idea of gender mainstreaming, but this and other issues that may be considered supplementary are allowable only when the original mandate of the donors has been met. It was within this allowable limit that NGO X was able to target issues of gender *ad hoc* through cash transfers and material goods to poor women, even though this was not a consistent practice or a holistic approach.

Ironically, the notion of gender mainstreaming originated from international development organizations; yet, as many scholars have argued, it is not always prioritized by these same vehicles of international development especially in the conduct of transnational health business, and as the evidence has shown.[48] Global policy commitment to gender issues and other social aspects of treatment are also reflected in the design of local programs. NGO X, which formerly managed the Erhoike health center, for example, cited dwindling and fluctuating funds as responsible for their *ad hoc* commitment to gender and other social considerations in treatment interventions. This particular claim, as prior analyses show, was attested to in the testimonies of HIV-seropositive women who access treatment at this facility. The initial claims of non-remuneration of salaries by the two HIV-seropositive women, leaders of the Courage HIV/AIDS support group at the Erhoike health center, were thus confirmed. A stakeholder in NGO X stated that specific funds allocated to this component of the treatment program were redirected to address the funder's objectives when the NGO experienced a funding shortfall from the donor.

> First of all, he who pays the piper dictates the tune, right? So if you are going to be using United States funds for our [local] programs, in as much as we will try to key along the rules of the country [Nigeria] we are working with, we will also have to uphold the rules of the United States Government as well, so issues that have to do with terrorism, race, gender and all were well addressed in our letter of agreement with our funders but when it comes to gender, our funding doesn't have any room specifically for gender issues or gender needs and all that.—Male NGO stakeholder

The salient point is that local commitment to gender mainstreaming in HIV/AIDS programs is partly a reflection of the inconsistencies in the global commitment to a gender priority, especially among international donors. The inconsistencies at this level are transferred to the local landscape through policies and programs as products of problematic alliances between NGOs and international development agencies, and which also foster new but intricate practices of development.

Donor influences and regulations also appear to vary by sector. As a policy maker noted, the public HIV/AIDS subsector mostly operates through bilateral partnerships with international funders but as an equal signatory and partner to agreements. In other words, funding relationships between international development agencies and public sector organizations are less regulated in the ways that funds are disbursed and allocated to specific issues compared to private sector organizations. Nevertheless, as this policy maker claimed, international funding agencies are now beginning to realize the importance of mainstreaming gender issues in development work but interest and commitment are mostly contingent on how naturalized these organizations are. That is, international development organizations with a strong local presence are better able to access firsthand knowledge of local gender issues and their significance, and thereby, enabling them to commit to redressing the issues.

Also significant to the ways that the global policy community impacts the local gender landscape is the transfer of specific standard international health norms and practices that inform how local HIV/AIDS institutions frame and practice gender in development. Most global health institutions have increasingly adopted a scientific approach to evaluate interventions.[49] This approach measures the performance and effectiveness of interventions on science-based universal methods that neglect the logic of assessing programs based on the specific needs, unique "practices and rationalities" of recipient countries.[50]

Global health programs often treat populations as homogenous entities when they frame and measure intervention impacts through purely quantitative measures, being overly preoccupied with statistics, for example, the rates of people with access to treatment but not the specific ways that individuals experience treatment.[51] Program assessments through the traditional monitoring and evaluation practices of international development agencies foreground sex-disaggregated data as a core method of assessment. Little attention is given to other confounding factors like social and economic class, marital status, and age, which differentiate experiences of specific populations. To illustrate with the experiences of HIV-seropositive women, the poor and uneducated ones were less likely to initiate treatment but more likely to drop out of treatment after initial uptake. Access and adherence to treatment were further complicated by age, as older women were found to be less consistent.

National and global statistics of ARV treatment in their current form, using sex-disaggregated data, thus, belie existing inequalities between and within gender groups that cannot be measured statistically. Yet, sex-disaggregated statistics remain the evaluative criteria designed to measure the impact of international development programs, including HIV/AIDS. Numeric measures of impact assessments negate a core principle of gender mainstreaming which is to assess the *implications* of particular policy actions on both women and men. A commonly used evaluation metric in international programs is the *impact indicator*, which like other indicators is operationalized quantitatively. Yet, technically, impact should be understood more comprehensively to include an outcome or change that is also qualitative. Although statistical counts may be cost-effective and less time-intensive, they negate a comprehensive approach to program assessments, especially if the goal of gender aimed for is transformative. In an assessment of the national gender response to the HIV/AIDS epidemic in Nigeria, conducted by NACA in 2013, qualitative data collection techniques, for example, focus group discussions, were deployed as gender assessment tools. Although time-consuming and cost-intensive, this produced a rich analysis of the national HIV/AIDS situation from a gender perspective. It assisted in unraveling where the national gender response was making substantive impact or otherwise.

In the final analysis, I also draw attention to how transnational relations shape local gender landscapes through knowledge transfer by way of capacity-building and training program content designed around Western development ideologies and practices that may not centralize local gender issues. Capacity-building programs have become a customary and staple component of local health governance with NGOs, especially mandated to continue this tradition as they implement donor-funded programs at the grassroots. Sometimes, trainers or mentors are foreign development actors. Even when they are indigenous, they have been trained by foreigners and thus utilize information accumulated from them. Again, these programs emphasize sex-disaggregated statistical data to measure and evaluate the impact of capacity-building.

Beyond the reductionism of program evaluation techniques is the categorical notion of gender that is constantly reproduced through global-local policy transfer with the erroneous assumption that gender equality means "gender balancing" using numbers. This is a false dichotomy between men and women, and which also erroneously conveys the notion that accomplishing gender equality is synonymous with having results of evaluations show parity in the numbers of men and women targeted or reached through interventions. Less emphasis is, therefore, on process and transformative development. Superficial impact measures obscure the relational power of gender and belie poverty, subordination, and other forms of oppression that women daily grapple within their micro-geographies. Yet, it is in this conscious deliberation and attention to (social) processes and context that the inequalities around women living with HIV can be reworked.

Gender mainstreaming in Nigerian HIV/AIDS interventions has run into the massive roadblocks of entrenched patriarchy and identity politics which make it to be situationally re-interpreted in a range of ways that sometimes assume gender means that women should be treated the same as men, and other times, that women need special treatment in order to come closer to equality with men. These have also produced tensions and conflicts among institutional actors, along gender lines.

Gender mainstreaming in this context also acts as a kind of prism that reveals the ways in which global health interventions and their institutionalized culture and practices fragment and split up developing countries' national health systems and any related systemic goal (like gender mainstreaming). Gender mainstreaming is thus fragmented and not practiced systematically across the landscape of HIV/AIDS interventions and it is also complicated in practice in the ways it is performed or elided in NGO programs to meet donor requirements for funding. For these reasons, gender mainstreaming in HIV/AIDS policies in Nigeria has remained a fancy and contested ideology that has gained some power in theory but not in practice.

Given this highly problematic context and the weight of structures that must be destabilized, gender mainstreaming may seem very idealistic and simplistic, even validating popular arguments on its limits. Still, gender mainstreaming can be a *concrete signifier* if it is backed by political will and if its true essence is understood as engendering positive and transformative change for both women and men.

NOTES

1. Doug Rosenberg and Matt Stephens, *Use Case Driven Object Modeling with UML: Theory and Practice* (Berkeley, CA: Apress, 2007), xxvii.

2. See Susanna Pinkus, "Bridging the Gap between Policy and Practice: Adopting a Strategic Vision for Partnership Working in Special Education," *British Journal of Special Education* 32, no. 4 (December 2005), https://doi.org/10.1111/j.1467-8578.2005.00395.x; Sally Shortall and Bettina Bock, "Introduction: Rural Women in Europe: The Impact of Place and Culture on Gender Mainstreaming the European Rural Development Programme," *Gender, Place and Culture: A Journal of Feminist Geography* 22, no. 5 (2015): 665, https://doi.org/10.1080/0966369X.2014.917819.

3. Public and private HIV/AIDS subsector policy stakeholders refer to individuals from HIV/AIDS institutions that operate under the government such as NACA and the FMoH, and local and international NGOs, respectively, all under the overall jurisdiction of the national health sector.

4. Nalia Kabeer, *Reversed Realities: Gender, Hierarchies in Development Thought* (London: Verso, 1994), xi. Also see Raewyn Connell, "Gender, Health and Theory: Conceptualizating the Issue in Local and World Perspective," *Social Science and Medicine* 74 (2012), https://doi.org/ 10.1016/j.socscimed.2011.06.006.

5. United Nations, *Report for the Economic and Social Council for 1997* (Geneva: United Nations Economic and Social Council, 1997), 3, http://www.un.org/womenwatch/daw/csw/GMS.PDF.

6. Margaret Alston, "Drought Policy in Australia: Gender Mainstreaming or Gender Blindness?" *Gender, Place and Culture: A Journal of Feminist Geography* 16, no. 2 (2009): 141, https://doi.org/10.1080/09663690902795738.

7. Ibid., 141.

8. Ibid.

9. Ibid.

10. Ibid. Also see United Nations, *Gender Mainstreaming. An Overview* (New York: United Nations, 2002), 1, http://www.un.org/womenwatch/osagi/pdf/e65237.pdf.

11. United Nations, *Report for the Economic and Social Council for 1997*, 3.

12. See United Nations Women, *Gender Mainstreaming in Development Programming: Guidance Note* (New York: United Nations Women, 2014), 7, https://undg.org/wp-content/uploads/2017/03/gender-mainstreaming-issuesbrief-en-pdf.pdf.

13. See ibid., 7; Greig et al., "Gender and AIDS: Time to Act," *AIDS* 22, suppl. 2 (August 2008): 3–4.

14. Cathy Mcllwaine and Kavita Datta, "From Feminizing to Engendering Development," *Gender, Place and Culture* 10, no. 4 (2003): 370–371, https://doi.org/10.1080/0966369032000155564.

15. Shortall and Bock, "Introduction: Rural Women in Europe," 663; Bettina B. Bock, "Gender Mainstreaming and Rural Development Policy: The Trivialization of Rural Gender Issues," *Gender, Place and Culture: A Journal of Feminist Geography* 22, no. 5 (2015): 731, https://doi.org/10.1080/0966369X.2013.879105.

16. George R. Glynis, "Interpreting Gender Mainstreaming by NGOs in India: A Comparative Ethnographic Approach," *Gender, Place and Culture: A Journal of Feminist Geography* 14, no. 6 (2007): 680, https://doi.org/1080/09663690701659143; Alston, "Drought Policy in Australia," 139.

17. Glynis, "Interpreting Gender Mainstreaming by NGOs in India," 680.

18. Ibid., 680.

19. See, for example, Kate Giles, *Pursuing Gender Equality Inside and Out* (Washington, DC: Population Reference Bureau, 2015), 10, 16.

20. See Jeneviève Mannell, "Conflicting Policy Narratives: Moving beyond Culture in Identifying Barriers to Gender Policy in South Africa," *Critical Social Policy* 34, no. 4 (2014): 455–457, https://doi.org/10.1177/0261018314538794.

21. Bock, "Gender Mainstreaming and Rural Development Policy," 732.

22. See Alston, "Drought Policy in Australia."

23. Bock, "Gender Mainstreaming and Rural Development Policy," 733.

24. See Shortall and Bock, "Introduction: Rural Women in Europe," 665; Glynis, "Interpreting Gender Mainstreaming by NGOs in India," 680.

25. Caroline Moser and Annalise Moser, "Gender Mainstreaming since Beijing: A Review of Success and Limitations in International Institutions," *Gender and Development* 13, no. 2 (July 2005): 15, https://doi.org/10.1080/13552070512331332283; Glynis, "Interpreting Gender Mainstreaming by NGOs in India," 680; Shortall and Bock, "Introduction: Rural Women in Europe," 663; Bock, "Gender Mainstreaming and Rural Development Policy," 731.

26. Glynis, "Interpreting Gender Mainstreaming by NGOs in India," 680–681; Bock, "Gender Mainstreaming and Rural Development Policy," 733.

27. Ibid., 733.

28. See Alston, "Drought Policy in Australia," 142; Bock, "Gender Mainstreaming and Rural Development Policy," 732.

29. See Kabeer, *Reversed Realities*.

30. Two NGOs were purposively selected for this investigation because of their direct affiliations with the Erhoike health center, for example, in the provision of HIV/AIDS resources, programmatic and technical assistance on ARV treatment as well as HIV care in this facility.

31. The GTC involves a cross section of individuals from national ministries, parastatals, and agencies such as the Ministry of Women Affairs, Ministry of Agriculture, and NACA, as well as international development agencies such as United Nations Women, United Nations Population Fund, and United Nations International Children's Emergency Fund, among others.

32. Vertical programs are disease-focused interventions that are deemed to be cost-effective but critics argue against their health exceptionalism approach which undermines an integrative or systems-wide approach to addressing diseases across a broader spectrum. For other references on vertical programs or selective disease interventions, see Marcos Cueto, "Origins of Primary Health Care and Selective Primary Health Care," *American Journal of Public Health* 94, no. 11 (November 2004); Julia A. Walsh and Kenneth S. Warren, "Selective Primary Health Care: An Interim Strategy for Disease Control in Developing Countries," *The New England Journal of Medicine* 30, no. 18 (1979).

33. See Glynis, "Interpreting Gender Mainstreaming by NGOs in India."

34. Alston, "Drought Policy in Australia," 141–142; Glynis, "Interpreting Gender Mainstreaming by NGOs in India," 680.

35. See Mannell, "Conflicting Policy Narratives," 458.

36. Ibid., 460.

37. Alston, "Drought Policy in Australia," 142.

38. See Fenella Porter and Caroline Sweetman, "Editorial," *Gender and Development* 13, no. 2 (July 2005): 2–4, https://doi.org/10.1080/13552070512331332283.

39. Alston, "Drought Policy in Australia," 150. Also see Shortall and Bock, "Introduction: Rural Women in Europe," 663.

40. Also see ibid.; George R. Glynis, "Interpreting Gender Mainstreaming by NGOs in India: A Comparative Ethnographic Approach," *Gender, Place and Culture: A Journal of Feminist Geography* 14, no. 6 (2007), https://doi.org/1080/09663690701659143.

41. Laurie Garrett, "The Challenge of Global Health," *Foreign Affairs* 86, no. 1 (January–February 2007): 23.

42. Ibid., 23.

43. For example, see Hakan Seckinelgin, "A Global Disease and Its Governance: HIV/AIDS in Sub-Saharan Africa and the Agency of NGOs," *Global Governance* 11, no. 3 (2005): 363.

44. See Pfeiffer et al., "Strengthening Health Systems in Poor Countries: A Code of Conduct for Nongovernmental Organizations," *American Journal of Public Health* 98, no. 12 (December 2008): 2135, https://doi.org/10.2105/AJPH.2007.125989.

45. Glynis, "Interpreting Gender Mainstreaming by NGOs in India," 682.

46. See Diana Mitlin, Sam Hickey, and Anthony Bebbington. "Reclaiming Development? NGOs and the Challenge of Alternatives," *World Development* 35, no. 10 (2007), https://doi.org/10.1016/j.worlddev.2006.11.005; Seckinelgin, "A Global Disease and Its Governance"; Bebbington, Anthony, "NGOs and Uneven Development: Geographies of Development Intervention," *Progress in Human Geography* 28, no. 6 (2004), https://doi.org/10.1191/0309132504ph516oa; Richa Nagar and Saraswati Raju, "Women, NGOs, and the Contradictions of Empowerment and Disempowerment: A Conversation," *Antipode* 35, no. 1 (February 2003), https://doi.org/10.1111/1467-8330.00298.

47. See Mitlin et al., "Reclaiming Development"; Seckinelgin, "A Global Disease and Its Governance"; Bebbington, "NGOs and Uneven Development: Geographies of Development Intervention."

48. Also see United Nations Women, *Gender Mainstreaming in Development Programming*, 7; United Nations, *Gender Mainstreaming*; Glynis, "Interpreting Gender Mainstreaming by NGOs in India," 681.

49. Giles, *Pursuing Gender Equality Inside and Out*, 15.

50. João Biehl, "When People Come First: Beyond Technical and Theoretical Quick-Fixes in Global Gealth," in *Global Political Ecology*, eds. Richard Peet, Paul Robbins, and Michael J. Watts (London: Routledge, 2011), 106.

51. Also see Sylvia H. Chant and Cathy McIlwaine, *Geographies of Development in the 21st Century: An Introduction to the Global South* (Cheltenham, UK: Edward Edgar, 2003), 218.

Chapter 10

Conclusion about an Unending Work

Throughout this book, the empirical evidence presented offers valuable insights into the proximate and global conditions in which women's unsustained HIV treatment access and adherence occur. The inadequacies of the biomedical model of health and health care in addressing social gaps in medicine, health, and well-being also make profound contributions to the health geography scholarship, which forms this book's main theoretical frame, as leading geographers continue to emphasize the need for social approaches to health over a monopoly of curative and scientific models.[1]

Importantly, the evidence also explains a proposition made earlier in this book, that is the paradox of free treatment yet unsustained access, attributed to institutional failures and poor gender representations at the level of policy and programs, among other factors. Through women's experiences of HIV treatment and self-reports of interventions, as well as policy discourses and analysis, effective representations of women and/or gender needs appear to be lacking in interventions. Current HIV treatment interventions are far divorced from the needs of women at the grassroots with inadequate interventions that fail to address women's social needs in treatment. As a result, HIV-seropositive women have made practical recommendations for more meaningful and participatory processes for them in both policy planning and formulation, such that these would allow them to vocalize their needs. In addition, this book also recommends a needs-right-based strategy that is deployed as an integrated framework to mainstream women's needs into development policies. This recommendation is not new whether in HIV/AIDS interventions in Nigeria or in traditional development practice.

Existing policy texts and discourses on HIV/AIDS interventions in Nigeria already deploy needs- and rights-based strategies, but they have not proven effective as, evidentially, current gaps remain in both treatment and other aspects of HIV/AIDS interventions. Yet the needs approach, when deployed effectively, offers a lot of potential in fulfilling the needs of intervention subjects, especially the poor, in development practice. Similarly, in contemporary development theory and practice, a strong needs strategy is often promoted and spoken of as a radical participatory approach to ensure meaningful involvement of the marginalized and grassroots population, including women, to define and control their own development needs.[2] On the other hand, the formalization and politicization of needs by development and aid agencies such that the subjects of development are stripped of their agency and direct involvement in development undermine a meaningful participatory approach.[3] This version of needs interpretation has been referred to as the weak needs approach.[4]

Given the silence of women in traditional development theory and practice, a rights-based approach was thus deployed to insert women into the development agenda in response to increased advocacy for women and gender considerations in development.[5] Especially in contemporary times, the rights-based approach has received greater advocacy among global and local feminists as paramount to improving the situation of women due to perceptions that the invocation of rights legitimizes the needs of women and thus ensures compliance by aid and development agencies.[6]

The needs-rights-based strategy is, however, hardly referenced as an integrated framework. Despite their inherent limitations, which this chapter explores through current HIV/AIDS interventions in Nigeria as well as this geography's sociocultural milieu, this chapter recommends the needs-rights-based strategy in its strongest form and as an integrative model to mainstream women and gender considerations in development. While the needs-based and rights-based approaches have their intrinsic merits, their benefits can only be maximized if their limitations are also duly addressed. Hence, I provide a cautionary tale that the merits of both approaches should not be taken *prima facie* as devoid of problems especially when deployed in specific spatial contexts. In this chapter, I clarify the specific ways that I recommend both approaches for a participatory gender framework and a more meaningful inclusion of women.

CLAIMING GENDER IN HEALTH THROUGH A NEEDS-RIGHTS APPROACH

In the feminist literature, the push for equality and women's emancipation has been increasingly premised on *rights* as rights provide the legal grounds to articulate and claim equal opportunities and access to resources for women.[7] In a world governed by the laws of patriarchy and where women's needs and interests have long been relegated, a rights-based approach is a particularly important tool to prioritize meeting women's basic needs and that of other vulnerable populations.[8] A needs-based approach, thus, derives its power and legitimacy by framing the fulfillment of basic needs which include services that ensure the health and well-being of individuals, as universal human rights within the United Nation's Universal Declaration of Human Rights framework.[9] It is in this sense that I argue that we cannot speak of needs in isolation of rights, just as it is in the same way that the exercise of rights and its entitlements are premised on particular needs, whether these are tangible or intangible resources. This forms a practical and theoretical basis for the needs-rights-based strategy to be viewed as an integrated framework in development theory and practice.

In the Nigerian context, equality, social justice, and rights are also key concepts that have been deployed to frame the discourse on women's emancipation particularly within the HIV/AIDS policy arena. Advocacy of women's rights has involved the identification of women's needs through consultations with representatives of people living with HIV/AIDS and gender experts at the national level, as the policy analysis revealed. While policy texts claimed the engagement of women living with HIV during policy planning and formulation at the national level, these were silent on the social demographics of women selected to represent the diverse categories of women living with HIV. Participation of local and poor women in policy discourses at the national level appeared to be lacking. Also related to this argument is the nature of *experts* or *gender consultants* that were solicited to identify and represent the needs of HIV-seropositive women in policy planning and formulation.

In traditional models of development that deploy the needs approach, women are rarely perceived to know what they need; instead, expert consultants and organizations are contracted to think and act on women's behalf especially in the needs identification process.[10] Traditional needs approach illuminates issues of power and representation such that the hierarchy of needs is top-down and not from the bottom-up. Although this can be argued to be remedied by subordinating *experts'* judgments to that of recipients, ambiguity of the nature of experts' representation, especially if the so-called experts are not fully informed in the local context, has adverse implications for policy implementation and outcomes, as well as the kinds of aid rendered to women.

I illustrate this argument with the Nigerian HIV/AIDS interventions. Although policies did not clearly state the nature of gender experts consulted for the inclusion of women into the policy planning process, there were indications that these were both local and foreign experts. I interviewed one such local gender expert whose responses revealed a vast knowledge of local gender issues, but like so many other institutional stakeholders, her class and social status color her gender lens. She levied undue power and agency for change upon local women and argued that the Nigerian woman should be able to "prove herself [and] double it," in the fight against male dominance and inequality. However, this level of presumed agency does not mirror the situations of HIV-seropositive women understudied, whose social and economic status weakly position them to fight against a system that is dominated by the men whom they feel emotionally, socially, and materially bound to and by men whom from all indications want to retain their power and privilege.

While I do comprehend the need for women to transition from the *passive* and *victim* statuses to active agents of change, there is a need to be deeply aware of individual social locations whether in terms of personal constraints, power, and privilege, and thus of poor women as such powerful agents of change. Simply put, knowledge of local gender issues matters in the needs identification process and as an important step within the needs-based approach but it is even more imperative for gender experts to be deeply aware and conscious of the ways that their social locations may influence their gender views and representation, as well as the social positions of the subjects they aim to represent.

Tensions around the degree of participation of development subjects, representation, and definition of *needs*, for example, who articulates needs, as well as the ways that development subjects are positioned within the needs framework, whether as activists or recipients, are some issues that make the traditional needs approach a basically flawed model of intervention.[11] These tensions have also come to delineate what is now termed the strong or radical needs approach and the weak needs approach within the basic needs framework.[12] The radical needs approach frames deprived subjects as active and the weak needs approach frames subjects of interventions as passive recipients.[13]

My proposition for the radical needs approach as an alternative to the traditional needs approach that is less participatory is not new but well-articulated in the development literature.[14] A meaningful and active participatory process is one that challenges the "politics of needs interpretation" from the perspectives of development subjects.[15] It is also an approach that operates under the principle that the subjects of interventions should be responsible for the identification and articulation of their needs, and control over their own lives and resources through collective and organized action aided by support groups.[16] In the Nigerian HIV/AIDS interventions, an alternative needs model should aim to move beyond a basic participatory and representative approach to a more direct and meaningful engagement of the subjects of interventions at all levels and not just the elite. Where gender experts are needed, they should be in direct consultation with all categories of HIV-seropositive women, irrespective of class and social locations—women who are most affected must be actively positioned and engaged within this framework.

One of the fundamental principles of human rights is the principle of nondiscrimination and inclusion in the access and ownership of liberties and entitlements. The focus here, however, is how this principle, if at all, informs public health policies on HIV treatment access and adherence. As have been argued in this book, the vulnerabilities of women living with HIV can be understood from a human rights perspective. Exposure and vulnerabilities to HIV transmission especially among women, in many sub-Saharan African spaces are produced from structural inequalities such as feminized poverty, oppression, and exploitation of women through social, cultural, and economic institutions that violate human rights. The United Nations convention on rights, thus, recognizes the fundamental need to protect minority groups and populations, and from this, the advocacy for women's rights to healthy living has emerged.

The 1948 United Nations Universal Declaration of Human Rights is part of a framework of declarations with significant legal and moral weight that include *the International Covenant on Economic, Social and Cultural Rights*, *the International Covenant on Civil and Political Rights*, and its *Optional Protocols*, under the auspices of the International Bill of Rights, a resolution of the United Nations General Assembly.[17] This framework also forms a part of the international customary law and has set the basis for other sub-laws at the international, regional, and national levels such as the *Convention of All Forms of Discriminations Against Women* (CEDAW) and the African Charter of Human Rights. But according to the United Nations Sustainable Development Partnership Framework, critical challenges remain among national institutions in the promotion and protection of human rights especially in their engagement with the United Nations human rights mechanism and the domestication of CEDAW which continues to be undermined by cultural and religious beliefs and practices (in Nigeria).[18] It is within this international legal framework that the claim for gender equity has been made within Nigeria's gender policy response to the HIV/AIDS epidemic.[19] Yet only minimal progress has been made in addressing the legal and human rights issues around the epidemic. And a number of reasons can be deduced.

Foremost is that, in Nigeria, policies do not automatically translate to law, meaning that they cannot be enforced in the courts of law. Evidently, institutional policy stakeholders attribute the weakness or failure to achieve an effective HIV/AIDS response to the non-legal backing of policies. While these sorts of narratives are commonplace in local policy discourses and in the legal scholarship that centers on HIV/AIDS and rights, I argue that the transformation of policies into laws is not the end to an existing weak legal response if the legal environment in which these policies are to be enacted as laws is flawed. However, I do share the popular opinion among policy stakeholders interviewed that when HIV/AIDS policies do not constitute law or embody the force and power of the law, they can be rendered weak and ineffective. Also, because policies are not legally binding on implementing institutions and partners, in practice, this eliminates the obligation to make recourse to policy guidelines. The engagement and effective implementation of HIV/AIDS policy guidelines are, therefore, left to the choice and will of implementing partners and may result in a selective and convenient application, given the lack of legally backed punitive measures as implied in the following policy statement.[20]

> They [HIV/AIDS policies] are merely administrative tools and guidelines that provide direction for governmental action. However, these policy documents can and may elaborate and specify the goals, values, and standards to which existing laws aspire and may be useful in interpreting the latter as well as guiding programmatic interventions by the government. . . . Currently, the 1999 Nigerian constitution and international treaties ratified by the country have provided the major sources of human rights for PLHIV and PABA in the country. However, as none of these treaties or the constitution specifically addresses the situation of PLHIV and PABA, the case of their applicability often has to be made through advocacy and lobbying. Thus, although PLHIV have human rights to be respected and protected, it is the tendency of the society to have pervasive prejudices and to overtly and covertly stigmatize and discriminate against PLHIV and PABA. A constitutional provision that does not speak HIV/AIDS contexts specifically does not do much to help the situation of the rights of PLHIV. And the protection of the rights of PLHIV and PABA are not on the priority radar screen of law enforcement agencies. The absence of explicit laws leaves PLHIV extremely vulnerable to the violation of their rights.

I argue, however, that even when policies on HIV/AIDS are ratified into laws, and invoked within a human rights perspective, they can also be contested or challenged by the meanings and interpretations assigned to these laws because rights emanate from and are contextualized by people's experiences.[21] For example, the African Charter of Human and People's Rights posits that "how human rights should be implemented and respected is a question of beliefs, values, solidarity, [and] organization strategies."[22] The Charter also articulates a rights-based approach that is reflective of historical traditions, local values, and beliefs.[23] Thus, the contextual interpretation and application of human rights may sometimes produce conflict with universal notions of rights. In Nigeria, this conflict is apparent in its mixed legal system comprising statutory, common, and traditional-religious laws (Sharia law is under this jurisprudence), the latter whose prescriptions sometimes differ from international conventions on human rights. CEDAW, for example, prohibits all forms of trafficking of women, exploitation of women and girls, and other forms of gender-based violence. Under the Sharia law, however, a female aged less than eighteen years is considered an adult when married—a law that exposes young adolescent women to intergenerational sex, male power, and control which are prerequisites for HIV transmission.

Also, under the common and Sharia laws, the criminal and penal code prescribe that a husband cannot be guilty of the offense of rape of his wife because unlawful carnal knowledge is defined as that which takes place otherwise than between a husband and a wife.[24] Women who go out of their way to seek redress for such acts become subject to the judgment of their character.[25] In other cases of gender-based violence, social power especially within intimate relationships and the pressure to conform to societal rules wield more power over the victims than the protective force of the law. A Nigerian woman who would seek redress from the law against her husband, for example, may be seen by her own family, peers, and the local and religious community as a betrayer because women are generally expected to protect their husband's reputation even when the men are at fault. It is a well-known fact in Nigeria that many cases of rape and domestic violence that happen within families when reported to the police have been waved off as a private and family matter, and therefore, should be settled as such. Although rights invoked through laws can serve as a protective force against social injustices, it does not automatically empower women or other vulnerable populations if those enacting the laws are not favorably disposed to making the law provide redress for those who seek it.

Demonstrably, human rights in the Nigerian context are intricately tied to existing structures of patriarchy and religious scripts. Among local women and men investigated for this research, the prescription of rights was invoked within cultural and religious mores. Women's rights have been framed along these lines and not within the notion of fundamental human rights. In a society like Nigeria where religious institutions and leaders are considered as bastions of power and authority, it is challenging to get people to be responsive against discriminatory religious practices. For example, religious organizations constantly violate rights to privacy and confidentiality through mandatory HIV/AIDS counseling and testing as a prerequisite for marriage in the church among intending couples.[26] Sometimes, employers and their organizations are also complicit in this violation of rights during employment and recruitment processes.[27] And it is within this flawed sociolegal environment that the rights for HIV vulnerable subjects have been proposed, pushed for, and practiced.

Thus, the overemphasis on the invocation of the human rights framework to achieve equity for vulnerable HIV subjects, although not entirely misplaced, does not necessarily translate to personal agency, redistributive power, and access to resources if the anomalies in the legal constitution and local contexts of rights are not challenged, reworked, and rewritten to equally favor women. Establishing rights is never the same as enacting or realizing them, and this reinforces a general criticism by scholars who propose a caution on the invocation of rights as absolute to resisting and redressing all inequalities.[28] Consequently, studies such as this that advocate for a rights-based approach also beckon on structural and transformative changes.[29]

A fundamental aim of this chapter is to elucidate the paradoxes, challenges, and dilemmas in the exercise of rights, as sometimes antithetical to its ideology. The deployment of human rights as a legal tool to frame needs and other forms of human entitlement is powerful but it is weak in application, in some contexts. While we may be quick to claim rights as the legal machinery to redress the subordination of marginalized women, the invocation of rights alone may be inadequate to deliver on the promises of freedom and equality if there is a lack of consciousness regarding its limitations because it loses its critical edge. In many instances, the notion of rights has been invoked as a token and mere rhetoric without the material agency and force of power needed to deliver what it claims.

This claim is not new as there are scholars who have argued that if rights do not necessarily transform the situation of women, why do we still make claims to rights as the *sine qua non* to women's freedom globally?[30] It is because "rights function to articulate a need, a condition of lack or injury"; otherwise our claims may lack any legitimacy if that need is not articulated or framed within a *rights* context.[31] A rights framework functions to legitimize women's needs in the fight for gender equality. It provides the necessary first step for which needs can be given agency and the basis to redress subsequent actions that may resist or stymie its enactment, and thereby, ensure that the opportunities, entitlements, and resources been claimed are actually channeled to the subjects of intervention. Karl Marx's analogous evaluation of rights to political emancipation articulates this poignantly that rights "certainly represent a great progress . . . not the final form of human emancipation . . . but [could be] the final form . . . within the framework of the prevailing social order."[32] Again, this speaks of the duality of rights in that its efficacy is spatially contingent yet it is a reality that is mostly unrecognized in studies that canvas heavily for this framework as instrumental for social justice.

What then are some practical and realizable solutions in articulating women's needs using a needs-right-based approach? A needs-based approach must be conscious of the politics of representation and popular interests which may be disconnected from the needs of recipients. It must always be mindful of whose conceptions of needs are deployed in interventions. HIV/AIDS policies on stigma and discrimination were translated into laws in Nigeria recently.[33] Yet it remains imperative to establish an enabling socio-legal environment for rights to be effectively claimed by the marginalized. Social education that is inclusive of gender awareness and male involvement remains key to troubling and reworking negative institutional and traditional mores as well as seeking redress for women's rights, and this must be centralized in HIV/AIDS policies.

FINAL NOTE

Our work starts where this book ends—as students, academic scholars, researchers, policy makers, and development actors. To begin with, the evidence from this book mandates a prioritization of context-specific HIV treatment interventions based on our knowledge of the complex personal politics, unique physical, and sociocultural and economic barriers that undermine access and adherence to ARTs among seropositive women in Nigeria's Niger Delta region.

Access and adherence to HIV treatment among poor and marginalized seropositive women in patriarchal settings are not at all linear as intervention maps may sometimes exemplify. Women who will initiate and consistently engage in treatment are those who have devised the means to first secure their basic needs and interests, which are mostly social in nature, as the evidence suggests that women place a stronger emphasis on the social body than the biological. The availability of free treatment is, thus, not always the primary motivator for initiating ARV access and maintaining adherence—a reality that demonstrates the need for health service access models to transcend the *availability* of health resources to underscoring the *types* of resources (whether social or biomedical, or both), as the latter has proved to be a stronger determinant of HIV treatment access and adherence in this context.

NOTES

1. See Vani S. Kulkarni and Subu V. Subramanian, "Social Perspectives on Health Inequalities," in *A Companion to Health and Medical Geography*, eds. Tim Brown, Sara McLafferty, and Graham Moon (Oxford: Wiley-Blackwell, 2010); Robin Kearns and Damian Collins, "Health Geography," in *A Companion to Health and Medical Geography*, eds. Tim Brown, Sara McLafferty, and Graham Moon (Oxford: Wiley-Blackwell, 2010); Mark Hunter, *Love in the Time of AIDS: Inequality, Gender and Rights in South Africa* (Bloomington: Indiana University Press, 2010).
2. Ben Wisner, *Power and Need in Africa* (Trenton: Africa World Press, 1982), 14.
3. Ibid., 14.
4. Ibid.
5. Cathy Mcllwaine and Kavita Datta, "From Feminizing to Engendering Development," *Gender, Place and Culture* 10, no. 4 (2003): 373, https://doi.org/10.1080/0966369032000155564.
6. Ibid.
7. See ibid.
8. Ben Wisner, *Power and Need in Africa* (Trenton: Africa World Press, 1982), 25.
9. See ibid., 25–26. Also see "Universal Declaration of Human Rights," United Nations, accessed November 12, 2018, http://www.un.org/en/universal-declaration-human-rights/.

10. Nalia Kabeer, *Reversed Realities: Gender, Hierarchies in Development Thought* (London: Verso, 1994), 230.

11. See Wisner, *Power and Need in Africa*, 27.

12. Ibid., 14.

13. Ibid.

14. Ibid., 15.

15. Kabeer, *Reversed Realities*, 230.

16. Ibid.

17. Gill Seidel, "The Competing Discourses of HIV/AIDS in Sub-Saharan Africa: Discourses of Rights and Empowerment and Discourses of Control and Exclusion," *Social Science and Medicine* 36, no. 3 (1993): 181.

18. United Nations, *Nigeria - United Nations Sustainable Development Partnership Framework (UNSDPF) 2018 to 2022* (Abuja: United Nations, 2017), 16, http://www.ng.undp.org/content/nigeria/en/home/library/knowledgeproducts/un-sustainable-development-partnership-framework-2018-2022.html.

19. For example, see National Agency for Food and Drug Administration and Control, *Gender Policy Handbook* (Abuja: National Agency for Food and Drug Administration and Control, 2014).

20. National Agency for the Control of AIDS, *National HIV/AIDS Strategic Plan 2010–2015* (Abuja: National Agency for the Control of AIDS, 2009), 21.

21. Also see Seidel, "The Competing Discourses of HIV/AIDS in Sub-Saharan Africa," 181.

22. Ibid.

23. "African (Banjul) Charter on Human and Peoples' Rights," accessed February 23, 2019, http://www.achpr.org/files/instruments/achpr/banjul_charter.pdf.

24. Eghosa Osa Ekhator, "Women and the Law in Nigeria: A Reappraisal," *Journal of International Women's Studies* 16, no. 2 (January 2015): 288.

25. Ibid., 288.

26. Also see Sambo Adamu Umar and Oche Mansur Oche, "Knowledge of HIV/AIDS and Use of Mandatory Premarital HIV Testing as a Prerequisite for Marriages among Religious Leaders in Sokoto, North Western Nigeria," *Pan African Medical Journal* 11, no. 27 (February 2012).

27. See "Implement HIV Workplace Policy, Anti-Discrimination Law, NACA Pleads," *Punch*, last modified May 1, 2018, https://punchng.com/implement-hiv-workplace-policy-anti-discrimination-law-naca-pleads/.

28. McIlwaine and Datta, "From Feminizing to Engendering Development," 374.

29. For example, see Greig et al., "Gender and AIDS: Time to Act," *AIDS* 22, no. 2 (August 2008), https://doi.org/10.1097/01.aids.0000327435.28538.18.

30. See Wendy Brown, "Suffering Rights as Paradoxes," *Constellations* 7, no. 2 (2000).

31. Ibid., 239.

32. Ibid.

33. See chapter 2, for a more detailed explanation of Nigeria's HIV/AIDS policies and legal framework.

Appendix

HIV/AIDS Policy Texts Analyzed

S/N	*Title of policy text*	*Responsible agency*	*Publication date*
1.	*HIV/AIDS in Nigeria, a USAID Brief*	United States Agency for International Development	2002
2.	*National Policy on HIV/AIDS*	National Agency for the Control of AIDS	2003
3.	*HIV/AIDS Emergency Action Plan 2001–2003/2004*	National Agency for the Control of AIDS	2001
4.	*HIV/AIDS National Strategic Framework for Action 2005–2009*	National Agency for the Control of AIDS and Society for Family Health	2005
5.	*National Guidelines for HIV and AIDS Treatment and Care in Adolescents and Adults by Federal Ministry of Health Abuja, Nigeria*	Federal Ministry of Health	2007
6.	*National Policy on HIV/AIDS*	National Agency for the Control of AIDS	2009
7.	*National HIV/AIDS Response Review 2005–2009*	National Agency for the Control of AIDS	2009
8.	*HIV/AIDS National Strategic Framework for Action 2010–2015*	National Agency for the Control of AIDS	2010
9.	*National Guidelines for HIV and AIDS Treatment and Care in Adolescents and Adults by Federal Ministry of Health Abuja*	Federal Ministry of Health	2010

(Continued)

(Continued)

S/N	Title of policy text	Responsible agency	Publication date
10.	*Women, Girls, Gender Equality and HIV. Five-Year Strategic Plan and Program Implementation Framework 2011–2015*	National Agency for the Control of AIDS	2011
11.	*Global AIDS Response: Country Progress Report Nigeria (GARPR)*	National Agency for the Control of AIDS	2012
12.	*Global AIDS Response: Country Progress Report Nigeria (GARPR)*	National Agency for the Control of AIDS	2014
13.	*Global AIDS Response: Country Progress Report Nigeria (GARPR)*	National Agency for the Control of AIDS	2015
14.	*Gender Assessment of the National Response to HIV/AIDS in Nigeria*	National Agency for the Control of AIDS	2013
15.	*Nigeria Operational Plan Report*	United States President's Emergency Plan for AIDS Relief	2013
16.	*National Guidelines on HIV/AIDS Care and Support*	National Agency for the Control of AIDS	2014
17.	*National Plan of Action: Addressing Gender-Based Violence and HIV/AIDS (GBV/HIV/AIDS) Intersections 2015–2017*	Federal Ministry of Women Affairs and Social Development	2014
18.	*Gender-Based Violence in Nigeria. National Guidelines and Referral Standards*	Federal Ministry of Women Affairs and Social Development	2014
19.	*Mapping of Laws, Policies and Services on Gender-Based Violence and Its Intersections with HIV in Nigeria*	National Agency for the Control of AIDS and United Nations Development Program	2014
20.	*Gender Policy Handbook*	National Agency for Food and Drug Administration and Control	2014
21.	*Global AIDS Response Country Progress Report*	National Agency for the Control of AIDS	2015
22.	*The Violence against Persons (Prohibition) Bill: An Analysis*	Choice for Life	N/A

Bibliography

Abdul, Mariam Marwa, Olayinka Adeleke, Olajumoke Adeyeye, Adenike Babalola, Emilia Eyo, Maryam Tauhida Ibrahim, Monica Voke-Ighorodje, and Martha Onose. *Analysis of the History, Organizations and Challenges of Feminism in Nigeria*. Spanish Agency for International Development Cooperation, 2012.

Abel, Emily K. and Margaret K. Nelson. "Circles of Care: An Introductory Essay." In *Circles of Care: Work and Identity in Women's Lives*, edited by Emily K. Abel and Margaret K. Nelson, 4–34. New York: State University of New York Press, 1990.

Acholonu, Catherine Obianuju. *Motherism: The Afrocentric Alternative to Feminism*. Owerri: Afa Publications, 1995.

Adebowale, Nike. "Nigeria: How Nigeria's 36 States Fare in HIV Prevalence." *Premium Times*, March 19, 2019. https://allafrica.com/stories/201903200030.html.

Aguwa, Jude. "Religion and HIV/AIDS Prevention in Nigeria." *Cross Currents*, 2 (2010): 208–223.

Aidoo, Ama Ata A. "Unwelcome Pals and Decorative Slaves - or Glimpses of Women as Writers and Characters in Contemporary African Literature." In *Literature and Society: Selected Essays on African Literature*, edited by Ernest Emeyonu, 17–37. Oguta: Zim Pan African Publishers, 1989.

Akeroyd, Anne V. "Coercion, Constraints, and 'Cultural Entrapments': A Further Look at Gendered and Occupational Factors Pertinent to the Transmission of HIV in Africa." In *HIV and AIDS in Africa: Beyond Epidemiology*, edited by Ezekiel Kalipeni, Susan Craddock, Joseph R. Oppong, and Jayati Ghosh, 89–103. Oxford: Blackwell, 2004.

Alston, Margaret. "Drought Policy in Australia: Gender Mainstreaming or Gender Blindness?" *Gender, Place and Culture: A Journal of Feminist Geography* 16, no. 2 (2009): 139–154. https://doi.org/10.1080/09663690902795738.

Aniekwu, Nkolika Ijeoma. "Converging Constructions: A Perspective on Sexuality and Feminism in Post-Colonial Africa." *African Sociological Review* 10, no. 1 (2006): 143–160.

Aniekwu, Nkolika Ijeoma. "Gender and Human Rights Dimensions of HIV/AIDS in Nigeria." *African Journal of Reproductive Health* 6, no. 3 (2002): 30–37.

Apostolova, Iva, and Elaina Gauthier-Mamaril. "Care and the Self: A Philosophical Perspective on Constructing Active Masculinities." *Feminist Philosophy Quarterly* 4, no. 1 (2018): 1–14. https://doi.org/10.5206/fpq/2018.1.2.

Arkell, Camille, and Mallory Harrigan, "HIV Treatment and an Undetectable Viral Load to Prevent HIV Transmission." CATIE. Last modified July 16, 2018. https://www.catie.ca/en/fact-sheets/transmission/hiv-viral-load-hiv-treatment-and-sexual-hiv-transmission.

Arndt, Susan. "African Gender Trouble and African Womanism: An Interview with Chikwenye Ogunyemi and Wanjira Muthoni." *Signs* 25, no. 3 (Spring 2000): 709–726.

Arndt, Susan. "Perspectives on African Feminism: Defining and Classifying African Feminist Literatures." *Agenda: Empowering Women for Gender Equity* 17, no. 54 (2002): 31–44. https://doi.org/10.1080/10130950.2002.9676176.

Bayer, Ronald. "Public Health Policy and the AIDS Epidemic: An End to HIV Exceptionalism?" *New England Journal of Medicine* 324, no. 21 (1991): 1500–1504.

Bebbington, Anthony. "NGOs and Uneven Development: Geographies of Development Intervention." *Progress in Human Geography* 28, no. 6 (2004): 725–745. https://doi.org/10.1191/0309132504ph516oa.

Biehl, João. "When People Come First: Beyond Technical and Theoretical Quick-Fixes in Global Gealth." In *Global Political Ecology*, edited by Richard Peet, Paul Robbins, and Michael J. Watts, 101–130. London: Routledge, 2011.

Billo, Emily and Nancy Hiemstra. "Mediating Messiness: Expanding Ideas of Flexibility, Reflexivity, and Embodiment in Fieldwork." *Gender, Place and Culture: A Journal of Feminist Geography* 20, no. 3 (2013): 313–328. https://doi.org/10.1080/0966369X.2012.674929.

Bock, Bettina B. "Gender Mainstreaming and Rural Development Policy: The Trivialization of Rural Gender Issues." *Gender, Place and Culture: A Journal of Feminist Geography* 22, no. 5 (2015): 731–745. https://doi.org/10.1080/0966369X.2013.879105.

Bor, Robert, Riva Miller, and Eleanor Goldman. "HIV/AIDS and the Family: A Review of Research in the First Decade." *Journal of Family Therapy* 15 (1993): 187–204.

Bowden, Peta. *Caring: Gender-Sensitive Ethics*. New York: Routledge, 1997.

Bressi, Sara K. and Elizabeth R. Vaden. "Reconsidering Self Care." *Clinical Social Work Journal* 45, no. 1 (2017): 33–38. https://doi.org/ 10.1007/s10615-016-0575-4.

British Broadcasting Corporation News. "Nigeria Leads in Religious Belief." Last modified February 26, 2004. http://news.bbc.co.uk/2/hi/programmes/wtwtgod/3490490.stm.

Brown, Wendy. "Suffering Rights as Paradoxes." *Constellations* 7, no. 2 (2000): 230–241.

Brown, Lisanne, Lea Trujillo, and Kate Macintyre. *Interventions to Reduce HIV/AIDS Stigma: What Have We Learned?* New Orleans: The Population Council, 2001.

Bryant, Raymond L. "Political Ecology. An Emerging Research Agenda in Third-World Studies." *Political Geography* 11, no. 1 (January 1992): 12–36.

Buve, Anne, Kizito Bishikwabo-Nzarhaza, and Gladys Mutangadura. "The Spread and Effect of HIV-1 Infection in Sub-Saharan Africa." *The Lancet* 359 (June 2002): 2011–2017.

Center for Laws of the Federation of Nigeria. "HIV/AIDS Anti-Discrimination Act 2014." Nigeria. Accessed September 11, 2018. http://lawnigeria.com/LawsoftheFederation/HIV-and-AIDS-%28Anti-Discrimination%29-Act,-2014.html.

Chant, Sylvia H. and Cathy McIlwaine. *Geographies of Development in the 21st Century: An Introduction to the Global South*. Cheltenham, UK: Edward Edgar, 2003.

Charmes, Jacques and Saskia Wieringa. "Measuring Women's Empowerment: An Assessment of the Gender-Related Development Index and the Gender Empowerment Measurement." *Journal of Human Development* 4, no. 3 (November 2003): 419–435. https://doi.org/10.1080/1464988032000125773.

Connell, Raewyn. "Gender, Health and Theory: Conceptualizating the Issue in Local and World Perspective." *Social Science and Medicine* 74 (2012): 1675–1683. https://doi.org/10.1016/j.socscimed.2011.06.006.

Craddock, Susan. "Beyond Epidemiology: Locating AIDS in Africa." In *HIV and AIDS in Africa: Beyond Epidemiology*, edited by Ezekiel Kalipeni, Susan Craddock, Joseph R. Oppong, and Jayati Ghosh, 1–10. Oxford: Blackwell, 2004.

Craddock, Susan. "Disease, Social Identity and Risk: Rethinking the Geography of AIDS." *Transactions of the Institute of British Geographers* 25, no. 2 (2000): 153–168.

Cueto, Marcos. "Origins of Primary Health Care and Selective Primary Health Care." *American Journal of Public Health* 94, no. 11 (November 2004): 1864–1874.

Dey, Soma, Bernadette P. Resurreccion, and Philippe Doneys. "Gender and Environmental Struggles: Voices from Adivasi Garo Community in Bangladesh." *Gender, Place and Culture* 21, no. 8 (2018): 945–962. https://doi.org/10.1080/0966369X.2013.832662.

Donovan, Courtney J. and Ian R. Duncan. "Situating Politics in Health and Medical Geography. In *A Companion to Health and Medical Geography*, edited by Tim Brown, Sara McLafferty, and Graham Moon, 173–223. Oxford: Wiley-Blackwell, 2010.

Dosekun, Simidele. "Defending Feminism in Africa." *Postamble* 3, no. 1 (2007): 41–47.

Drabek, Anne G. "Development Alternatives: The Challenge for NGOs - an Overview of the Issues." *World Development* 15 (1987): ix–xv.

Dyck, Isabel. "Feminism and Health Geography: Twin Tracks or Divergent Agendas?" *Gender, Place and Culture* 10, no. 4 (December 2003): 361–368. https://doi.org/10.1080/0966369032000153331.

Dyck, Isabel and Parin Dossa. "Place, Health and Home: Gender and Migration in the Constitution of Healthy Space." *Health and Place* 13 (2007): 691–701. https://doi.org/10.1016/j.healthplace.2006.10.004.

Edwin, Bernard J. "Nigeria: Senate Passes Law Criminalizing HIV Non-Disclosure, Exposure and Transmission with Vague and Overly Broad Statute." HIV Justice Network. Last modified June 4, 2015. http://www.hivjustice.net/news/nigeria-senate-passes-law-criminalising-hiv-non-disclosure-exposure-and-transmission-with-vague-and-overly-broad-statutes-in-the-sexual-offences-bill/.

Ekhator, Eghosa Osa. "Women and the Law in Nigeria: A Reappraisal." *Journal of International Women's Studies* 16, no. 2 (January 2015): 285–296.

Eller, Cynthia. *The Myth of Matriachal Prehistory: Why an Invented Past Wont Give Women a Future*. Boston, MA: Beacon Press, 2000.

Escobar, Arturo. "Histories of Development, Predicaments of Modernity: Thinking about Globalization from Some Critical Development Studies Perspective." In *Rural Transformation and Development - China in Context: The Everyday Lives of Policies and People*, edited by Norman Long, Ye Jingzhong, and Wang Yihuan, 25–53. Cheltenham, UK: Edward Elgar, 2010.

European Institute for Gender Equality. "Female-headed Households." Gender Equality Glossary and Thesaurus. Accessed February 9, 2019. https://eige.europa.eu/rdc/thesaurus/terms/1126.

Exploring Your Mind. "Self-Care Is a Sign of Freedom, Says Michel Foucault." Psychology. Last modified November 14, 2017. https://exploringyourmind.com/self-care-sign-freedom-says-michel-foucault/.

Ezeigbo, Akachi. *Snail-Sense Feminism: Building on an Indigenous Model*. Lagos: University of Lagos, 2012.

Faria, Caroline. "Privileging Prevention, Gender Responsibility: An Analysis of the Ghanaian Campaign against AIDS." *Social and Cultural Geography* 9, no. 1 (February 2008): 41–70. https://doi.org/10.1080/14649360701789584.

Farmer, Paul. *AIDS and Accusation: Haiti and the Geography of Blame*. Berkeley: University of California Press, 1992.

Farmer, Paul. *Infections and Inequalities. The Modern Plagues*. Berkeley: University of California Press, 1999.

Farmer, Paul. *Pathologies of Power*. Berkeley: University of California Press, 2005.

Farmer, Paul E., Bruce Nizeye, Sara Stulac, and Salmaan Keshavjee. "Structural Violence and Clinical Medicine." *PLoS Medicine* 3, no. 10 (October 2006): 1686–1691. https://doi.org/10.1371/journal.pmed.0030449.

Fisher, Berenice and Joan C. Tronto, "Toward a Feminist Theory of Care." In *Circles of Care: Work and Identity in Women's Lives*, edited by Emily K. Abel and Margaret K. Nelson, 35–62. New York: State University of New York Press, 1990.

Fisher, William A., Taylor Kohut, and Jeffrey D. Fisher. "AIDS Exceptionalism: On the Social Psychology of HIV Prevention Research." *Social Issues Policy Review* 3, no. 1 (December 2009): 1–29. https://doi.org/10.1111/j.1751-2409.2009.01010.x.

Floyd, Sian, Amelia C. Crampin, Judith R. Glynn, Michael Mwenebabu, Stancelaus Mnkhondia, Bagrey Ngwira, Basia Zaba, and Paul E. M. Fine. "The Long Term Social and Economic Impact of HIV on the Spouses of Infected Individuals in Northern Malawi." *Tropical Medicine and International Health* 13, no. 4 (2008): 520–531. doi:10.1111/j.1365–3156.2008.02030.x.

Forman, Lisa. "Global AIDS Funding and the Re-Emergence of AIDS 'Exceptionalism'." *Social Medicine* 6, no. 1 (2011): 45–51.

Foucault, Michel. *Subjectivity and Truth Ethics: Subjectivity and Truth*. New York: The New Press, 1997.

Frye, Victoria, Princess Fortin, Sonja Mackenzie, David Purcell, Lorece V. Edwards, Shannon Gwinn Mitchell, Eduardo Valverde, R. Garfein, Lisa Metsch, and Mary H. Latka. "Managing Identity Impacts Associated with Disclosure of HIV Status: A Qualitative Investigation." *AIDS Care: Psychological and Socio-Medical Aspects of AIDS/HIV* 21, no. 8 (2009): 1071–1078. https://doi.org/10.1080/09540120802657514.

Garcia, María-Cristina Díaz and Friederike Welter. "Gender Identities and Practices: Interpreting Women's Entrepreneurs' Narratives." *International Small Business Journal* 31, no. 4 (June 2013): 384–404. https://doi.org/10.1177/0266242611422829.

Gardner, Daniel K. *The Four Books: The Basic Teachings of the Later Confucian Tradition*. Indianapolis, IN: Hackett Publishing Company Inc., 2007.

Garrett, Laurie. "The Challenge of Global Health." *Foreign Affairs* 86, no. 1 (January–February 2007): 14–38.

Geng, Elvin. "Retention in Care for HIV-Infected Patients in Resource-Limited Settings: Challenges and Opportunities." HIV InSite. Last modified January, 2011. http://hivinsite.ucsf.edu/InSite?page=md-expert-geng.

Gesler, Wilbert M. "Therapeutic Landscapes: Theory and a Case Study of Epidauros, Greece." *Environment and Planning Development: Society and Space* 11 (1993): 171–189.

Giles, Kate. *Pursuing Gender Equality Inside and Out*. Washington, DC: Population Reference Bureau, 2015.

Gilligan, Carol. "Carol Gilligan." Ethics of Care. Last modified June 16, 2011. http://ethicsofcare.org/carol-gilligan/.

Gilligan, Carol. *In a Different Voice: Psychological Theory and Women's Development*. Cambridge, MA: Harvard University Press, 1982.

Glynis, George R. "Interpreting Gender Mainstreaming by NGOs in India: A Comparative Ethnographic Approach." *Gender, Place and Culture: A Journal of Feminist Geography* 14, no. 6 (2007): 679–701. https://doi.org/1080/09663690701659143.

GNP+. *HIV Leadership through Accountability Programme: GNP+, NEPWHAN. PLHIV Stigma Index Nigeria Country Assessment*. Amsterdam: GNP+, 2011. http://www.stigmaindex.org/sites/default/files/reports/Nigeria%20StigmaIndex%20final_HighRs.pdf.

Greig, Alan, Dean Peacock, Rachel Jewkes, and Sisonke Msimang. "Gender and AIDS: Time to Act." *AIDS* 22, suppl. 2 (August 2008): 1–14. https://doi.org/10.1097/01.aids.0000327435.28538.18.

Griffin, Penny. "The World Bank, HIV/AIDS and Sex in Sub-Saharan Africa: A Gendered Analysis." *Globalizations* 8, no. 2 (April 2011): 229–248.

Goffman, Erving. *Stigma: Notes on the Management of Spoiled Identity*. Englewood Cliffs, NJ: Prentice Hall, 1963.

Golden-Timstar, Rebecca. "Amnesty and New Violence in the Niger Delta." Forbes. Last modified March 20, 2018. https://www.forbes.com/sites/uhenergy/2018/03/20/amnesty-and-new-violence-in-the-niger-delta/#7188c1d7263f.

Hankivsky, Olena. "Women's Health, Men's Health and Gender and Health: Implications of Intersectionality." *Social Science and Medicine* 74 (2012): 1712–1720. https://doi.org/ 10.1016/j.socscimed.2011.11.029.

Haraway, Donna. "Situated Knowledges: The Science Question in Feminism and the Privilege of Partial Perspective." *Feminist Studies* 14, no. 3 (Fall 1988): 575–599.

Hardin, Marie and Erin Whiteside. "From Second-Wave to Poststructuralist Feminism." *Evolving Frameworks for Viewing Women's Sports* 5 (2012): 1–21.

Harvey, David. *A Brief History of Neoliberalism*. New York: Oxford University Press, 2005.

Hawkes, Sarah J. and Kent Buse. "Gender and Global Health: Evidence, Policy and Inconvenient Truths." *The Lancet* 381 (2013): 1783–1787.

Held, Virginia. *The Ethics of Care: Personal, Political, and Global*. New York: Oxford University Press, 2006.

Herek, Gregory M., Leonard Mitnick, Scott Burris, Margaret Chesney, Patricia Devine, Mindy Thompson Fullilove, Robert Fullilove, Herbet Chao Gunther, Jeffrey Levi, and Stuart Michaels. "Workshop Report: AIDS and Stigma: A Conceptual Framework and Research Agenda." *AIDS and Public Policy Journal* 13, no. 1 (Spring 1998): 36–47.

Hodgson, Ian. "Empathy, Inclusion and Enclaves: The Culture of Care of People with HIV/AIDS and Nursing Implications." *Issues and Innovations in Nursing Practice* 55, no. 3 (2006): 283–290. https://doi/10.1111/j.1365-2648.2006.03913.x.

Huairou Commission. *Uniting Communities around Caregiving: Grassroots Women's Perspectives on the HIV/AIDS Pandemic: A Report from the Grassroots Women's International Academy and YWCA International Women's Summit, Nairobi, Kenya*. Brooklyn, NY: Huairou Commission, 2007. https://huairou.org/wp-content/uploads/2016/06/Huairou_YWCA_Report.pdf.

Hunter, Mark. *Love in the Time of AIDS: Inequality, Gender and Rights in South Africa*. Bloomington: Indiana University Press, 2010.

Imam, Ayesha M. "The Dynamics of WINning: An Analysis of Women in Nigeria (WIN)." In *Feminist Genealogies, Colonial Legacies, Democratic Futures*, edited by M. Jacqui Alexander and Chandra Talpade Mohanty, 280–307. New York: Routledge, 1997.

International Labor Organization. *ABC of Women Workers' Rights and Gender Equality*. Geneva: International Labor Organization, 2007. http://www.ilo.org/wcmsp5/groups/public/---dgreports/---gender/documents/publication/wcms_087314.pdf.

Inyang, Emem Bassey and Ekaete Evans Udong. "Livelihood Insecurity and Diversification among Women in an Environmentally Challenged Niger Delta Region, Nigeria." *The International Journal of Humanities and Social Science* 1, no. 1 (2013): 44–52.

Jarosz, Lucy. "Constructing the Dark Continent: Metaphor as Geographic Representation of Africa." *Geografiska Annaler. Series B, Human Geography* 74, no. 2 (1992): 105–115.

Kabeer, Nalia. "Gender Equality and Women's Empowerment: A Critical Analysis of the Third Millennium Development Goal." *Gender and Development* 13, no. 1 (March 2005): 13–24. https://doi.org/10.1080/13552070512331332273.

Kabeer, Nalia. *Reversed Realities: Gender, Hierarchies in Development Thought.* London: Verso, 1994.

Kalofonos, Ippolytos. "'All I Eat Is ARVs': The Paradox of AIDS Treatment Interventions in Central Mozambique." *Medical Anthropology Quarterly* 24, no. 3 (2010): 363–380. https://doi.org/ 10.1111/j.1548–1387.2010.01109.x.

Kearns, Robin. "The Place of Health in the Health of Place: The Case of Hokianga Special Medical Area." *Social Science and Medicine* 33 (1991): 519–530.

Kearns, Robin and Damian Collins. "Health Geography." In *A Companion to Health and Medical Geography*, edited by Tim Brown, Sara McLafferty, and Graham Moon, 15–32. Oxford: Wiley-Blackwell, 2010.

Kearns, Robin and Graham Moon. "From Medical to Health Geography: Novelty, Place and Theory after a Decade of Change." *Progress in Human Geography* 26, no. 5 (2002): 605–625. https://doi.org/10.1191/0309132502ph389oa.

Kevane, Michael. *Women and Development in Africa: How Gender Works*. Boulder, CO: Lynne Rienner, 2004.

Kolawole, Mary Modupe. "Transcending Incongruities: Rethinking Feminism and the Dynamics of Identity in Africa." *Agenda: Empowering Women for Gender Equity* 17, no. 54 (2002): 92–98. https://doi.org/10.1080/10130950.2002.9676183.

Kolawole, Mary Modupe. *Womanism and African Consciousness*. Eritrea: Africa World Press, 1997.

Krishnan, Suneeta, Megan S. Dunbar, Alexandra Minnis, Carol A. Medlin, Caitlin E. Gerdts, and Nancy S. Padian. "Poverty, Gender Inequities, and Women's Risk of Human Immunodeficiency Virus/AIDS." *Annals of the New York Academy of Sciences* 1136 (2008): 101–110. https://doi.org/10.1196/annals.1425.013.

Kulkarni, Vani S. and Subu V. Subramanian. "Social Perspectives on Health Inequalities." In *A Companion to Health and Medical Geography*, edited by Tim Brown, Sara McLafferty, and Graham Moon, 375–398. Oxford: Wiley-Blackwell, 2010.

Lawson, Victoria. "Geographies of Care and Responsibility." *Annals of the Association of American Geographers* 97, no. 1 (2007): 1–11.

Lazzarini, Zita. "What Lessons Can We Learn from the Exceptionalism Debate (Finally)?" *Journal of Law, Medicine and Ethics* 29, no. 2 (2001): 149–151.

Liamputtong, Pranee, Niphattra Haritavorn, and Niyada Kiatying-Angsulee. "HIV and AIDS, Stigma and AIDS Support Groups: Perspectives from Women Living with HIV and AIDS in Central Thailand." *Social Science and Medicine* (2009): 1–7. https://doi.org/10.1016/j.socscimed.2009.05.040.

Lugalla, Joe L. P. "The Impact of Structural Adjustment Policies on Women's and Children's Health in Tanzania." *Review of African Political Economy* 22, no. 63 (March 1995): 43–53.

Lurie, Peter, Percy Hintzen, and Robert A. Lowe. "Socioeconomic Obstacles to HIV Prevention and Treatment in Developing Countries: The Roles of the International Monetary Fund and the World Bank." In *HIV and AIDS in Africa: Beyond Epidemiology*, edited by Ezekiel Kalipeni, Susan Craddock, Joseph R. Oppong, and Jayati Ghosh, 204–212. Oxford: Blackwell, 2004.

Lyttleton, Chris. "Fleeing the Fire: Transformation and Gendered Belonging in Thai HIV/AIDS Support Groups." *Medical Anthropology: Cross Cultural*

Studies in Health and Illness 23, no. 1 (2004): 1–40. https://doi/10.1080/0145 9740490275995.

Madunagu, Bene E. "The Nigerian Feminist Movement: Lessons from Women in Nigeria, WIN." *Review of African Political Economy* 35, no. 118 (2008): 666–673.

Makaudze, Godwin. "Empowerment or Delusion?: The Shona Novel and Women Emancipation." *Journal of Literary Studies* 32, no. 1 (2016): 70–83. https://doi.org /10.1080/02564718.2016.1158985.

Mannell, Jenevième. "Conflicting Policy Narratives: Moving beyond Culture in Identifying Barriers to Gender Policy in South Africa." *Critical Social Policy* 34, no. 4 (2014): 454–474. https://doi.org/10.1177/0261018314538794.

Marshall, Don D. "The New World Group of Dependency Scholars." In *The Companion to Development Studies*, edited by Vandana Desai and Robert B. Potter, 184–190. London: Routledge, 2014.

Mayer, Jonathan. "The Geographical Understandings of HIV/AIDS in Sub-Saharan Africa." *Norwegian Journal of Geography* 59 (2005): 6–13. https://doi.org/ 10.1080/00291950510020493.

Mayer, Jonathan and Melinda S. Meade. "A Reformed Medical Geography Reconsidered." *The Professional Geographer* 46, no. 1 (February 1994): 103–106.

Mbire-Barungi, Barbara. "Ugandan Feminism: Political Rhetoric or Reality?" *Women's Studies International Forum* 22, no. 4 (1999): 435–439.

McCarthy, Jane Ribbens. "The Powerful Relational Language of 'Family': Togetherness, Belonging and Personhood." *The Sociological Review* 60, no. 1 (2012): 68–90.

Mcllwaine, Cathy and Kavita Datta. "From Feminizing to Engendering Development." *Gender, Place and Culture* 10, no. 4 (2003): 369–382. https://doi.org/10.1080/096 6369032000155564.

Medecins Sans Frontiers. *Out of Focus: How Millions of People in West and Central Africa Are Being Left Out of the Global HIV Response*. Medecins Sans Frontiers, 2016. https://www.msf.org/sites/msf.org/files/2016_04_hiv_report_eng.pdf.

Medina, José. *Speaking from Elsewhere: A New Contextualist Perspective Meaning, Identity and Discursive Agency*. Albany: State University of New York Press, 2006.

Mercer, Claire. "NGOs, Civil Society and Democratization: A Critical Review of the Literature." *Progress in Development Studies* 2, no.1 (2002): 5–22. https://doi.org/ 10.1191/1464993402ps027ra.

Mitlin, Diana, Sam Hickey, and Anthony Bebbington. "Reclaiming Development? NGOs and the Challenge of Alternatives." *World Development* 35, no. 10 (2007): 1699–1720. https://doi.org/10.1016/j.worlddev.2006.11.005.

Moser, Caroline and Annalise Moser. "Gender Mainstreaming since Beijing: A Review of Success and Limitations in International Institutions." *Gender and Development* 13, no. 2 (July 2005): 11–22. https://doi.org/10.1080/13552070512331332283.

Mountz, Alison and Jennifer Hyndman. "Feminist Approaches to the Global Intimate." *Women's Studies Quarterly* 34, no. 1/2 (Spring 2006): 446–463.

Nagar, Richa and Saraswati Raju. "Women, NGOs, and the Contradictions of Empowerment and Disempowerment: A Conversation." *Antipode* 35, no. 1 (February 2003): 1–13. https://doi.org/10.1111/1467-8330.00298.

Nasidi, Abdulsalami and Tekena O. Harry. "The Epidemiology of HIV/AIDS in Nigeria." In *AIDS in Nigeria: A Nation on the Threshold*, edited by O. Adeyi, P. J. Kanki, O. Odutolu, and J. A. Idoko, 17–36. Cambridge, MA: Harvard Center for Population and Development Studies, 2006.

National Agency for Food and Drug Administration and Control. *Gender Policy Handbook*. Abuja: National Agency for Food and Drug Administration and Control, 2014.

National Agency for the Control of AIDS. *Global AIDS Response: Country Progress Report, Nigeria*. Abuja: National Agency for the Control of AIDS, 2015. http://www.unaids.org/sites/default/files/country/documents/NGA_narrative_report_2015.pdf.

National Agency for the Control of AIDS. *Global AIDS Response: Country Progress Report. Nigeria GARPR 2014*. Abuja: National Agency for the Control of AIDS, 2014.

National Agency for the Control of AIDS. *HIV/AIDS Emergency Action Plan 2001–2003/2004*. Abuja: National Agency for the Control of AIDS, 2001.

National Agency for the Control of AIDS. *HIV/AIDS National Strategic Framework for Action 2005–2009*. Abuja: Society for Family Health, 2005.

National Agency for the Control of AIDS. *HIV/AIDS National Strategic Framework for Action Plan 2010–2015*. Abuja: National Agency for the Control of AIDS, 2010.

National Agency for the Control of AIDS. *National Guidelines on HIV/AIDS Care and Support*. Abuja: National Agency for the Control of AIDS, 2014.

National Agency for the Control of AIDS. *National HIV/AIDS Response Review*. Abuja: National Agency for the Control of AIDS, 2009.

National Agency for the Control of AIDS. *National HIV and AIDS Strategic Framework 2017–2021*. Abuja: National Agency for the Control of AIDS, 2017. https://www.childrenandaids.org/sites/default/files/2017-11/NATIONAL-HIV-AND-AIDS-STRATEGIC-FRAMEWORK.pdf.

National Agency for the Control of AIDS. *National HIV/AIDS Strategic Plan 2010–2015*. Abuja: National Agency for the Control of AIDS, 2009.

National Agency for the Control of AIDS. *National Policy on HIV/AIDS*. Abuja: National Agency for the Control of AIDS, 2003.

National Agency for the Control of AIDS. *National Policy on HIV/AIDS*. Abuja: National Agency for the Control of AIDS, 2009.

Network of People Living with HIV/AIDS in Nigeria. "Network of People Living with HIV and AIDS in Nigeria (NEPWHAN)." About Us. Accessed February 15, 2019. http://nepwhan.net/?page=About-Us.

Network of People Living with HIV/AIDS in Nigeria. *HIV and AIDS Work Place Policy*. Abuja: Network of People Living with HIV/AIDS in Nigeria, 2013. http://nepwhan.net/assets/policy_HIV_Work_Place_Policy_June_2013.pdf.

Network of People Living with HIV/AIDS in Nigeria. *Financial Policy and Procedural Manual*. Abuja: Network of People Living with HIV/AIDS in Nigeria, 2013.

Niger Delta AIDS Response. *Establishing and Sustaining HIV Comprehensive Care Services in Cottage Hospitals in the Niger Delta: Report of the Niger Delta AIDS Response Project*. Abuja: Family Health International, 2009.

Nkealah, Naomi. "(West) African Feminisms and Their Challenges." *Journal of Literary Studies* 32, no. 2 (2016): 61–74. https://doi/org/10.1080/02564718.2016.|1198156.

Nnaemeka, Obioma. "Nego-feminism: Theorizing, Practicing and Pruning Africa's Way." *Signs: Journal of Women in Culture and Society* 29, no. 2 (2003): 357–385.

Nthabiseng, Phaladze and Sheila Tlou. "Gender and HIV/AIDS in Botswana: A Focus on Inequalities and Discrimination." *Gender and Development* 14, no. 1 (2006): 23–35. https://doi.org/10.1080/13552070500518095.

Ntozi, James P. M. and Samuel Zirimenya. "Changes in Household Composition and Family Structure during the AIDS Epidemic in Uganda." *The Continuing African HIV/AIDS Epidemic* (1999): 193–209.

Nyambedha, Erick Otieno, Simiyu Wandibba, and Jens Aagaard-Hansen. "Changing Patterns of Orphan Care Due to the HIV Epidemic in Western Kenya." *Social Science and Medicine* 57 (2003): 301–311.

Odeyemi, Isaac A. O. and John Nixon. "Assessing Equity in Health Care through the National Health Insurance Schemes of Nigeria and Ghana: A Review-Based Comparative Analysis." *International Journal for Equity in Health* 12, no. 9 (2013): 1–18.

Ogundipe-Leslie, Molara. *Re-Creating Ourselves: African Women and Critical Transformations*. Trenton, NJ: Africa World Press, 1994.

Ojanuga, Durrenda Nash and Cathy Gilbert. "Women's Access to Health Care in Developing Countries." *Social Science and Medicine* 35, no. 4 (1992): 613–617.

Okoko, Eno. "Women and Environmental Change in the Niger Delta, Nigeria: Evidence from Ibeno." *Gender Place and Culture* 6, no. 4 (1999): 373–378. https://doi.org/10.1080/09663699924944.

Okoli, Al Chukwuma. "The Political Ecology of the Niger Delta Crisis and the Prospects of Lasting Peace in the Post-Amnesty Period." *Global Journal of Human Social and Political Science* 13, no. 3 (2013): 37–46.

Olarinmoye, Omobolaji O. "Faith-Based Organizations and Development: Prospects and Constraints." *Transformation: An International Journal of Holistic Mission Studies* 29, no. 1 (2012): 1–14. https://doi.org/10.1177/0265378811427985.

Oluduro, Oluwole. "The Role of Religious Leaders in Curbing the Spread of HIV/AIDS in Nigeria." *Potchefstroom Electronic Law Journal* 13, no. 3 (2010): 205–236.

Onyekwere, Joseph. "HIV/AIDS Anti-Discrimination Law and Essence of Implementation." *The Guardian*. Last modified April 14, 2015. https://guardian.ng/features/law/hivaids-anti-discrimination-law-and-essence-of-implementation/.

Oppenheimer, Gerald M. and Ronald Bayer. "The Rise and Fall of AIDS Exceptionalism." *American Medical Association Journal of Ethics* 11, no. 12 (2009): 988–992.

Oyekanmi, Felicia Durojaiye. "Institutionalization of Gender Inequality in Nigeria: Implications for the Advancement of Women." *Population Review* 44, no. 1 (2005): 56–71. https://doi.org/10.1353/prv.2005.0005.

Para-Mallam, Oluwafunmilayo Josephine. "Faith, Gender and Development Agendas in Nigeria: Conflicts, Challenges, and Opportunities." *Gender and Development* 14, no. 3 (2007): 409–421. https://doi.org/10.1080/13552070600980898.

Paudel, Vikas and Kedar P. Baral. "Women Living with HIV/AIDS (WLHA), Battling Stigma, Discrimination and Denial and the Role of Support Groups as a Coping Strategy: A Review of Literature." *Reproductive Health* 12, no. 53 (2015): 1–18. https://doi/10.1186/s12978-015-0032-9.

People's Health Movement, Medact, and Global Equity Gauge Alliance. *Global Health Watch 2: An Alternative World Health Report*. London: Zed Books, 2008.

Pfeiffer, James, Wendy Johnson, Meredith Forth, Aaron Shakow, Amy Hagopian, Steve Gloyd, and Kenneth Gimbel-Sherr. "Strengthening Health Systems in Poor Countries: A Code of Conduct for Nongovernmental Organizations." *American Journal of Public Health* 98, no. 12 (December 2008): 2134–2140. https://doi.org/10.2105/AJPH.2007.125989.

Pinkus, Susanna. "Bridging the Gap between Policy and Practice: Adopting a Strategic Vision for Partnership Working in Special Education." *British Journal of Special Education* 32, no. 4 (December 2005): 184–187. https://doi.org/10.1111/j.1467-8578.2005.00395.x.

Plazy, Mélanie, Joanna Orne-Gliemann, François Dabis, and Rosemary Dray-Spira. "Retention in Care Prior to Antiretroviral Treatment Eligibility in Sub-Saharan Africa: A Systematic Review of the Literature." *BMJ Open* 5 (2015): 1–10. https://doi.org/10.1136/bmjopen-2014–006927.

Policy Brief. *Access Challenges for HIV Treatment among People Living with HIV and Key Populations in Middle-Income Countries* (2013). https://msmgf.org/wp-content/uploads/2015/09/Access_Challenges_for_HIV_treatment_KAPs.pdf.

Porter, Elisabeth. "Rethinking Women's Empowerment." *Journal of Peacebuilding and Development* 8, no. 1 (July 2013): 1–14. https://doi.org/10.1080/15423166.2013.785657.

Porter, Fenella and Caroline Sweetman. "Editorial." *Gender and Development* 13, no. 2 (July 2005): 2–10. https://doi.org/10.1080/13552070512331332283.

Punch. "Implement HIV Workplace Policy, Anti-Discrimination Law, NACA Pleads." Last modified May 1, 2018. https://punchng.com/implement-hiv-workplace-zpolicy-anti-discrimination-law-naca-pleads/.

Ramjee, Gita and Brodie Daniels. "Women and HIV in Sub-Saharan Africa." *AIDS Research and Therapy* 10, no. 30 (December 2013): 1–9. https://doi.org/10.1186/1742-6405-10-30.

Reda, Ayalu A. and Sibhatu Biadgilign. "Determinants of Adherence to Antiretroviral Therapy among HIV-Infected Patients in Africa." *AIDS Research and Treatment* 2012 (February 2012): 574–656. https://doi.org/10.1155/2012/574656.

Reuters. "Nigeria Opens 41 New AIDS Treatment Centers." Last modified March 14, 2006. http://www.aegis.org/news/re/2006/RE060316.html.

Ricketts, Thomas C. "Accessing Health Care." In *A Companion to Health and Medical Geography*, edited by Tim Brown, Sara McLafferty, and Graham Moon, 521–539. Oxford: Wiley-Blackwell, 2010.

Robinson, Fiona. *The Ethics of Care: A Feminist Approach to Human Security*. Philadelphia, PA: Temple University Press, 2011.

Rose, Nikolas. "The Politics of Life Itself." *Theory, Culture and Society* 18, no. 6 (December 2001): 1–30.

Rosenberg, Doug and Matt Stephens. *Use Case Driven Object Modeling with UML: Theory and Practice*. Berkeley, CA: Apress, 2007.

Rosenberg, Mark W. and Kathleen Wilson. "Remaking Medical Geography." *Territoris* 5 (2005): 17–32.

Rosenberg, Tina. "Look at Brazil." *New York Times*, 26–63, January 28, 2001.

Rosenbrock, Rolf, Francois Dubois-Arber, Martin Moers, Patrice Pinell, Doris Schaeffer, and Michel Setbon. "The Normalization of AIDS in Western European Countries." *Social Science and Medicine* 50 (2000): 1607–1629.

Roy, Arundhati. "The NGO-ization of Resistance." *Toward Freedom*. Last modified September 8, 2014. http://www.towardfreedom.com/33-archives/globalism/3660-arundhati-roy-the-ngo-ization-of-resistance.

Schoepf, Brooke Grundfest. "AIDS, History, and Struggles over Meaning." In *HIV and AIDS in Africa: Beyond Epidemiology*, edited by Ezekiel Kalipeni, Joseph R. Oppong, and Jayati Ghosh, 15–28. Oxford: Blackwell, 2004.

Schwartländer, Bernhard, Ian Grubb, and Jos Perriëns. "The 10-Year Struggle to Provide Antiretroviral Treatment to People with HIV in the Developing World." *Lancet* 368 (August 2006): 541–546.

Seckinelgin, Hakan. "A Global Disease and Its Governance: HIV/AIDS in Sub-Saharan Africa and the Agency of NGOs." *Global Governance* 11, no. 3 (2005): 351–368.

Seeley, Janet, Rachel Grellier, and Tony Barnett. "Gender and HIV/AIDS Impact Mitigation in Sub-Saharan Africa: Recognizing the Constraints." *Journal of Social Aspects of HIV/AIDS* 1, no. 2 (August 2004): 87–98.

Seidel, Gill. "The Competing Discourses of HIV/AIDS in Sub-Saharan Africa: Discourses of Rights and Empowerment and Discourses of Control and Exclusion." *Social Science and Medicine* 36, no. 3 (1993): 175–194.

Setel, Phillip. *A Plague of Paradoxes: AIDS, Culture and Demography in Northern Tanzania*. Chicago: University of Chicago Press, 2000.

Shortall, Sally and Bettina Bock. "Introduction: Rural Women in Europe: The Impact of Place and Culture on Gender Mainstreaming the European Rural Development Programme." *Gender, Place and Culture: A Journal of Feminist Geography* 22, no. 5 (2015): 662–669. https://doi.org/10.1080/0966369X.2014.917819.

Sidaway, James D. "Post-Development." In *The Companion to Development Studies*, edited by Vandana Desai and Robert B. Potter, 227–234. London: Routledge, 2014.

Simon, E. D. "The Niger Delta Region and the Woman's Predicament: A Study of Kaine Agary's *Yellow Yellow*." *African Research Review* 4, no. 3b (July 2010): 155–166.

Skoe, Eva E. and Rhett Diessner. "Ethic of Care, Justice, Identity, and Gender: An Extension and Replication." *Merrill-Palmer Quarterly* 40, no. 2 (April 1994): 272–289.

Smith, Julia H. and Alan Whiteside. "Exceptional Epidemics: AIDS Still Deserves a Global Response." *Globalization and Health* 5, no. 15 (2009): 1–8.

Sparke, Matthew. "Health." In *The SAGE Handbook of Progress in Human Geography*, edited by Roger Lee, Noel Castree, Rob Kitchin, Vicky Lawson, Anssi Paasi, Sarah Radcliffe, and Charles Withers, 684–708. Thousand Oaks, CA: Sage, 2014.

Springer, Kristen W., Jeanne M. Stellman, and Rebecca M. Jordan-Young. "Beyond a Catalogue of Differences: A Theoretical Frame and Good Practice Guidelines for Researching Sex/Gender in Human Health." *Social Science and Medicine* 74 (2012): 1817–1824. https://doi.org/10.1016/j.socscimed.2011.05.033.

Springer, Kristen W., Olena Hankivsky, and Lisa M. Bates. "Gender and Health: Relational, Intersectional, and Biosocial Approaches." *Social Science and Medicine* 74, no. 11 (March 2012): 1661–1666. https://doi.org/10.1016/j.socscimed.2012.03.001.

Thompson, Linda. "Conceptualizing Gender in Marriage: The Case of Marital Care." *Journal of Marriage and Family* 55, no. 3 (August 1993): 557–569.

Tong, Rosemarie. "The Ethics of Care: A Feminist Virtue Ethics of Care for Healthcare Practitioners." *Journal of Medicine and Philosophy* 23, no. 2 (1998): 131–152.

Tronto, Joan. *Moral Boundaries: A Political Argument for a Ethic of Care*. New York: Routledge, 1993.

Udoh, Isidore. "Oil, Migration, and the Political Economy of HIV/AIDS Prevention in Nigeria's Niger Delta." *International Journal of Health Services* 43, no. 4 (2013): 681–697. https://doi.org/10.2190/HS.43.4.f.

Umar, Sambo Adamu and Oche Mansur Oche. "Knowledge of HIV/AIDS and Use of Mandatory Premarital HIV Testing as a Prerequisite for Marriages among Religious Leaders in Sokoto, North Western Nigeria." *Pan African Medical Journal* 11, no. 27 (February 2012).

UNAIDS. *Access to Antiretroviral Therapy in Africa: Status Report on Progress towards the 2015 Targets*. Geneva: UNAIDS, 2013. http://www.unaids.org/sites/default/files/media_asset/20131219_AccessARTAfricaStatusReportProgresstowards2015Targets_en_0.pdf.

UNAIDS. "AIDS Info: Nigeria." Accessed August 8, 2019, http://aidsinfo.unaids.org/.

UNAIDS. "Country Factsheets: Nigeria, 2017." Data. Accessed July 16, 2018. http://www.unaids.org/en/regionscountries/countries/nigeria.

UNAIDS. "Nigeria Passes Law to Stop Discrimination Related to HIV." Update. Last modified February 11, 2015. http://www.unaids.org/en/resources/presscentre/featurestories/2015/february/20150211_nigeria_law.

UNAIDS. "Nigeria: Progress towards 90-90-90 Target." Accessed July 31, 2019. http://aidsinfo.unaids.org/.

UNAIDS. *"Three Ones" Key Principles: "Coordination of National Responses to HIV/AIDS," Guiding Principles for National Authorities and Their Partners*. Geneva: UNAIDS, 2004. http://data.unaids.org/una-docs/three-ones_keyprinciples_en.pdf.

UNAIDS. *UNAIDS Data 2019*. Geneva: UNAIDS, 2019. https://www.unaids.org/sites/default/files/media_asset/2019-UNAIDS-data_en.pdf.

United Nations. *Gender Mainstreaming. An Overview*. New York: United Nations, 2002. http://www.un.org/womenwatch/osagi/pdf/e65237.pdf.

United Nations. "International Widow's Day, 23 June." Accessed September 14, 2018. http://www.un.org/en/events/widowsday/.

United Nations. *Nigeria - United Nations Sustainable Development Partnership Framework (UNSDPF) 2018 to 2022*. Abuja: United Nations, 2017. http://www.ng.undp.org/content/nigeria/en/home/library/knowledgeproducts/un-sustainable-development-partnership-framework-2018-2022.html.

United Nations. *Report for the Economic and Social Council for 1997*. Geneva: United Nations Economic and Social Council, 1997. http://www.un.org/womenwatch/daw/csw/GMS.PDF.

United Nations. *Widowhood: Invisible, Secluded or Excluded*. Geneva: United Nations Division for the Advancement of Women, 2001. http://www.un.org/womenwatch/daw/public/wom_Dec%2001%20single%20pg.pdf.

United Nations. *The World's Women 2015: Trends and Statistics*. New York: United Nations Department of Economic and Social Affairs, 2015. https://unstats.un.org/unsd/gender/downloads/worldswomen2015_report.pdf.

United Nations. "Universal Declaration of Human Rights." Accessed November 12, 2018. http://www.un.org/en/universal-declaration-human-rights/. United Nations Development Program. *Niger Delta Human Development Report*. Abuja: United Nations Development Program, 2006.

United Nations Women. *Gender Mainstreaming in Development Programming: Guidance Note*. New York: United Nations Women, 2014. https://undg.org/wp-content/uploads/2017/03/gender-mainstreaming-issuesbrief-en-pdf.pdf.

United Nations Women. "Statement: Widows Rights to Independent Life and Livelihood after Loss." Last modified June 21, 2017. http://www.unwomen.org/en/news/stories/2017/6/statement-un-women-international-widows-day.

United Nations World Food Program (WFP). *HIV/AIDS Analysis: Integrating HIV/AIDS in Food Security and Vulnerability Analysis*. Rome: Vulnerability Analysis and Mapping Branch and HIV/AIDS Service, 2008. https://documents.wfp.org/stellent/groups/public/documents/manual_guide_proced/wfp193482.pdf.

United States Agency for International Development. *HIV/AIDS in Nigeria: A USAID Brief*. Abuja: United States Agency for International Development, 2002.

van den Berg, Wessel, Kirsty Brittain, Gareth Mercer, Dean Peacock, Kathryn Stintson, Hanna Janson, and Vuyiseka Dubula. "Improving Men's Participation in Preventing Mother-to-Child Transmission of HIV as a Maternal, Neonatal, and Child Health Priority in South Africa." *PloS Medicine* 12, no. 4 (April 2015): 1–8. https://doi.org/10.1371/journal.pmed.1001811.

Vlassoff, Carol and Claudia Garcia Moreno. "Placing Gender at the Center of Health Programming: Challenges and Limitations." *Social Science and Medicine* 54 (2002): 1713–1723.

Walsh, Julia A. and Kenneth S. Warren. "Selective Primary Health Care: An Interim Strategy for Disease Control in Developing Countries." *The New England Journal of Medicine* 30, no. 18 (1979): 967–974.

Watts, Michael. "Antimonies of Community: Some Thoughts on Geography, Resources, and Empire." *Transactions of the Institute of British Geography* 29, no. 2 (2004): 195–216.

Watts, Michael. "Resource Curse? Governmentality, Oil and Power in the Niger Delta, Nigeria." *Geopolitics* 9, no. 1 (2004): 50–80. https://doi.org/10.1080/14650040412331307832.

Watts, Michael. "Righteous Oil? Human Rights, the Oil Complex and Corporate Social Responsibility." *Annual Review of Environment and Resources* 30 (July 2005): 9.1–9.35. https://doi.org/10.1146/annurev.energy.30.050504.144456.

Weinberg, Merlinda. "The Ideological Dilemma of Subordination of Self versus Self-Care: Identity Construction of the 'Ethical Social Worker'." *Discourse and Society* 25, no. 1 (2014): 84–99. https://doi.org/ 10.1177/0957926513508855.

Wisner, Ben. *Power and Need in Africa.* Trenton, NJ: Africa World Press, 1982.

World Health Organization. *Consolidated Guidelines on the Use of Antiretroviral Drugs for Treating and Preventing HIV Infection.* Geneva: World Health Organization, 2013. https://www.who.int/hiv/pub/guidelines/arv2013/operational/en/.

World Health Organization. "Faith-Based Organizations Play a Major Role in HIV/AIDS Care and Treatment in Sub-Saharan Africa." Last modified February 8, 2007. http://www.who.int/mediacentre/news/notes/2007/np05/en/.

World Health Organization. "Three Ones Agreed by Donors and Developing Countries." The 3 by 5 Initiative. Accessed January 14, 2019. https://www.who.int/3by5/newsitem9/en/.

World Health Organization. "Viral Suppression for HIV Treatment Success and Prevention of Sexual Transmission of HIV." HIV/AIDS. Accessed February 19, 2019. https://www.who.int/hiv/mediacentre/news/viral-supression-hiv-transmission/en/.

World Health Organization and Joint United Nations Program on HIV/AIDS. *Guidance on Provider-Initiated HIV Testing and Counselling in Health Facilities.* Geneva: World Health Organization and Joint United Nations Program on HIV/AIDS, 2007. https://www.who.int/hiv/pub/guidelines/9789241595568_en.pdf.

Wright, Melissa W. "Geography and Gender: Feminism and a Feeling of Justice." *Progress in Human Geography* 34, no. 6 (2010): 818–827. https://doi.org/10.1177/0309132510362931.

Index

Page references for figures are italicized

About the Author

Eloho Ese Basikoro is the founder and president of BATOP Research and Consulting Services, and has more than 10 years of professional experience in research, teaching, and international development in multinational contexts. She holds a doctorate degree in health and medical geography from the University of Washington, Seattle.

Lightning Source UK Ltd.
Milton Keynes UK
UKHW040400031219
354417UK00001BB/44/P

9 781786 607706